OXFORD MEDICAL PUBLICATIONS

Cardiovascular Disease in the Elderly

Cardiovascular Disease in the Elderly

A Practical Manual

Rosaire Gray

Consultant Physician and Honorary Senior Lecturer at UCL,
Department of Cardiovascular Medicine,
Whittington Hospital,
London, UK

Louise Pack

Consultant Physician, Medicine for the Elderly,
Brighton and Sussex University Hospitals Trust,
Brighton, UK

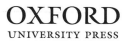

OXFORD
UNIVERSITY PRESS

OXFORD
UNIVERSITY PRESS

Great Clarendon Street, Oxford OX2 6DP

Oxford University Press is a department of the University of Oxford.
It furthers the University's objective of excellence in research, scholarship,
and education by publishing worldwide in

Oxford New York

Auckland Cape Town Dar es Salaam Hong Kong Karachi
Kuala Lumpur Madrid Melbourne Mexico City Nairobi
New Delhi Shanghai Taipei Toronto

With offices in

Argentina Austria Brazil Chile Czech Republic France Greece
Guatemala Hungary Italy Japan Poland Portugal Singapore
South Korea Switzerland Thailand Turkey Ukraine Vietnam

Oxford is a registered trade mark of Oxford University Press
in the UK and in certain other countries

Published in the United States
by Oxford University Press Inc., New York

British Library Cataloguing in Publication Data
Data available

Library of Congress Cataloging-in-Publication-Data
Data available

Typeset by Glyph International, Bangalore, India
Printed in Great Britain
on acid-free paper by
Ashford Colour Press Ltd., Gosport, Hampshire

ISBN 978–0–19–957059–1

10 9 8 7 6 5 4 3 2 1

Foreword

It is predicted that by 2033, in the United Kingdom, those aged 65 and over will be twenty-three percent of the total population and 3.2 million will be aged 85 and over.

As we know, cardiovascular disease is becoming more common with increasing age and currently there are insufficient cardiologists to provide the care exclusively in this country.

Strategies need to be formulated to approach the challenge of the managing this major health issue. Geriatricians, general practitioners, specialist cardiac nurses both in secondary and primary care and other healthcare professionals need to be able to be able to confront and feel confident to provide the necessary care for the condition.

This book is therefore a timely publication. Its authors set out, with clarity, a neatly systematic approach in general to the management of cardiovascular disease in the elderly, with additional information on dealing with relevant, pertinent issues related to the age group. The chapters are well laid out with useful, clear diagrams and well organised tables together with a summary of important points to remember, references, and a recommended reading list. Latest clinical trials are succinctly mentioned and with guidelines, including those from the National Institute for Health and Clinical Excellence (NICE).

The management, involving relevant medication, of a range of cardiovascular conditions is included together with a very useful chapter on elderly cardiac patients undergoing non cardiac surgery. Also addressed in separate sections are issues of co-morbidity, particularly mental health, and medical treatment and the approach of end of life.

This publication sets out to be a practical manual and there is no doubt that in the fourteen chapters, the authors have admirably achieved their objective. The book should be essential reading for consultants, general practitioners, specialist nurses, medical students and healthcare professionals both in the community and in hospital. I am very happy to recommend this book and heartily congratulate the authors who have tackled a very pressing current challenge with an excellent approach.

Dr. Simon M. Wiseman MBBS FRCGP
Programme Director
Primary Care Education
Whittington Education Centre.
Whittington Hospital

Foreword

Preface

Demographic changes have led to an increasing number of older people needing healthcare, and cardiovascular diseases are particularly prevalent in the elderly. The healthcare needs of the elderly often differ from those of younger patients as their needs are often more complex, in view of the physical, psychological, and social changes associated with ageing, as well as the presence of other co-morbidities. Older people may present atypically, are more vulnerable to therapeutic delays or errors, and the response to treatment may alter with ageing and presence of other co-morbidities.

Traditionally elderly care medicine is multidisciplinary and the care of the older person with cardiovascular disease requires input from many professions including cardiologists, cardiothoracic surgeons, care of the elderly physicians, primary care doctors, specialist nurses, pharmacists, and other professions allied to medicine. This book should appeal to all of these as well as junior doctors in training.

With advances in therapy (medical, surgical, and devices), the prognosis of most cardiovascular conditions has improved, but the elderly have traditionally not been included in clinical trials and are often not considered for these therapies when they become available.

This book aims to cover as comprehensively as possible how to manage elderly patients with common cardiovascular conditions. The overall aim is to provide simple, clear advice on diagnosis, investigation, and treatment options available with special reference to the elderly population.

We have endeavoured to give as contemporary and up-to-date view as possible of management of cardiovascular disease in the elderly. However, we recognize that the pace of publication and progress can and often does overtake the speed of publication. This is a first edition and we recognize it is not perfect, and we would invite feedback and recommendations for the future.

Contents

Detailed contents

Contributors

Ruth Law
ST4 Geriatrics/GIM, Whittington Hospital,
London, UK
(Chapter 5: Heart failure, and Chapter 13: Medical treatment
and approaching end of life)

Gareth Rosser
ST1 Core Medical Trainee, Whittington Hospital,
London, UK
(Chapter 6: Arrhythmias)

Abbreviations

AAA	abdominal aortic aneurysm
ABPM	ambulatory blood pressure measurement
ABPI	ankle brachial pressure index
ACE	angiotensin-converting enzyme
AChE	acetylcholinesterase
ACP	advance care planning
ACS	acute coronary syndrome
AF	atrial fibrillation
AR	aortic regurgitation
ARB	angiotensin receptor II blocker
AS	aortic stenosis
ASD	atrial septal defect
AT	atrial tachycardia
AV	atrioventricular
AVNRT	atrioventricular nodal re-entrant tachycardia
AVR	aortic valve replacement
AVRT	atrioventricular re-entrant tachycardia
BBB	bundle branch block
bd	twice daily
BMI	body mass index
BNP	brain natriuretic peptide
BP	blood pressure
CABG	coronary artery bypass graft
CCF	chronic/congestive heart failure
CGA	comprehensive geriatric assessment
CHB	(complete) heart block
CHD	coronary heart disease
CK	creatinine kinase
COPD	chronic obstructive pulmonary disease
CRT	cardiac resynchronization therapy
CSH	coronary sinus hypersensitivity
CSH	carotid sinus hypersensitivity
CSM	carotid sinus massage
CT	computed tomography
CXR	chest radiograph
DAT	dual antiplatelet therapy

DBP	diastolic blood pressure
DOLS	deprivation of liberty safeguards
ECG	electrocardiogram
EMI	electromagnetic interference
ESC	European Society of Cardiology
GFR	glomerular filtration rate
HBPM	home blood pressure monitoring
HDL	high-density lipoprotein
HDU	high dependency unit
HR	heart rate
ICD	implantable cardioverter-defibrillator
IHD	ischaemic heart disease
IMCA	independent mental capacity advocate
INR	international normalized ratio
ISDN	isosorbide dinitrate
ISH	isolated systolic hypertension
ITU	intensive care unit
JVP	jugular venous pressure
LA	left atrium
LAD	left anterior descending artery
LBBB	left bundle branch block
LCP	Liverpool Care Pathway
LMWH	low molecular weight heparin
LPA	Lasting Power of Attorney
LV	left ventricular
LVEF	left ventricular ejection fraction
LVF	left ventricular failure
LVH	left ventricular hypertrophy
MAT	multifocal atrial tachycardia
MCA	Mental Capacity Act
METs	metabolic equivalent of activities of daily living
MI	myocardial infarction
MMSE	Mini-Mental State Examination
MR	mitral regurgitation
MRI	magnetic resonance imaging
MS	mitral stenosis
NHS	National Health Service
NSTEMI	non-ST segment elevation myocardial infarction
NT-proBNP	N-terminal pro-BNP
NYHA	New York Heart Association

od	once daily
PAF	paroxysmal atrial fibrillation
PCI	percutaneous coronary intervention
PPP	proton pump inhibitor
prn	at night
PVD	peripheral vascular disease
qds	four times daily
QoL	Quality of Life
rtPA	recombinant tissue plasminogen activator
RV	right ventricle
SA	sinoatrial
SAQ	Seattle Angina questionnaire
SBP	systolic blood pressure
SNRI	serotonin-norepinephrine reuptake inhibitor
SR	sinus rhythm
SSRI	selective serotonin reuptake inhibitor
ST	sinus tachycardia
STEMI	ST segment elevation myocardial infarction
SVT	supraventricular tachycardia
TAVI	transcatheter aortic valve replacement
TCA	tricyclic antidepressant
tds	three times daily
TIA	transient ischaemic attack
TIMI	Thrombolysis in Myocardial Infarction
TR	tricuspid regurgitation
TSH	thyroid-stimulating hormone
U+Es	urea and electrolytes
VT	ventricular tachycardia

Chapter 1

The ageing population

Demographics

- The UK population is ageing rapidly.
- Between 1983 and 1998, there was an increase of 1.5 million people aged 65 and over; this age group now accounts for 16% of the UK population and is predicted to account for 23% of the UK population by 2033.
- The fastest growing age group is the 'oldest old', those aged 85 years and over. This group is predicted to more than double in number from 1.3 million in 1998 (2% of the population) to 3.2 million in 2033, continuing the previous rise from 0.6 million in 1983.
- The population of centenarians is predicted to increase by 7% per year (Fig. 1.1).

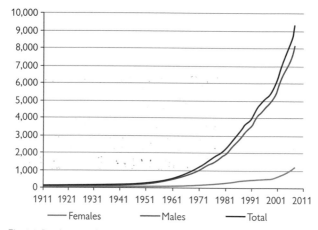

Fig. 1.1 Population aged 100 years and over, as at 1 January 2009, England and Wales (from National Statistics online (www.statistics.gov.uk). Reproduced under the terms of the Click-Use licence).

Increased survival is due to a number of factors, including improvements in medical treatment, hygiene, sanitation, nutrition, and living standards. More recently, mortality improvements have been greater in the male population, so the current ratio of female to male centenarians is expected to fall. In view of these demographic changes, it is increasingly important for healthcare professionals to know about the management of cardiovascular disease in elderly patients in order to provide the best quality care.

Issues for the future

Cardiovascular disease becomes increasingly common with age. Keeping up with the evidence base is difficult. In the UK we do not have enough cardiologists, so many elderly patients with cardiovascular disease are looked after by geriatricians and general practitioners. Ageism is still a problem and the elderly are often not referred for appropriate investigation and treatment due to lack of awareness of advances in cardiology that apply to older people. Cardiologists, geriatricians, general practitioners and other healthcare professionals need to work more closely to ensure better evidence-based and multidisciplinary care for the growing population of elderly people.

Effects of ageing on the heart

The effects of ageing on the heart result in a reduced threshold for clinical expression of common cardiac diseases in the elderly, such as atrial fibrillation (AF) and chronic heart failure. Ageing can also impact on the clinical manifestations and prognosis of these diseases.

- Left ventricular wall thickness – increases progressively with age, even in people without cardiovascular disease. The increase is due to increase in average myocyte size, although myocyte numbers decrease. Increased impedance to left ventricular ejection (due to reduced arterial compliance) also contributes to left ventricular hypertrophy.
- Ventricular stiffness – increases due to interstitial fibrosis and collagen. Associated with decreased ventricular relaxation.
- Left ventricular filling and preload – by the age of 80, the diastolic filling rate has reduced by 50% compared with that of a 20-year-old heart. As a result, more filling occurs in late diastole, which requires more vigorous atrial contraction. Hence the haemodynamic consequences of atrial fibrillation are often more significant in the elderly.
- Atrial enlargement – occurs due to more vigorous atrial contraction. May result in a fourth heart sound.
- Left ventricular ejection – the end-systolic volume regulation begins to fail with advancing age, resulting in deteriorating regulation of the ejection fraction.
- Stroke volume – is maintained in normal healthy individuals but as a result of reduced heart rate response to exercise, cardiac output reserve decreases by about 30% between the ages of 20 and 85 years. Hence, the cardiac index can increase by only about 2.5-fold in an older person compared with 3.5-fold in a younger person.
- Heart rate – there is no difference in resting supine heart rate between older and younger people. However, there is a reduction in the variations that occur with respiration (heart rate ↓ on expiration) due to autonomic changes with ageing.
- Cardiac output – as heart rate reserve falls with advancing age, so does cardiac output (see above).
- Sinoatrial node – reduction in pacemaker cells, and the number and sensitivity of β-receptors, leads to a reduction of intrinsic and maximal sinus rate. For example, when exercising, the maximum heart rate is reduced by a third between the ages of 20 and 85. The older heart therefore relies on increased stroke volume to increase cardiac output when exercising (see above).
- Fibrosis of the conducting system – increases the risk of bundle branch block and/or complete heart block.
- Thickening of heart valves due to calcification and fibrosis – associated with minor degrees of valvular dysfunction in healthy elderly people. Aortic sclerosis may give rise to systolic murmur, but no significant pressure gradient.
- Deposition of amyloid intracellularly in the myocardium and walls of small coronary arteries – present in 80–100% of older people at post mortem, although the majority do not develop symptoms of amyloid cardiomyopathy.
- Circulating catecholamines increase.

Effects of ageing on blood vessels

(See Fig. 1.2.)

- Aorta and major arteries elongate and stiffen with thickening of smooth muscle in the arterial wall. Leads to increased systolic blood pressure and increased pulse wave velocity.
- Reduction in arterial baroreceptor sensitivity may result in orthostatic hypotension.
- Decreased endothelial function.
- Atherosclerosis.

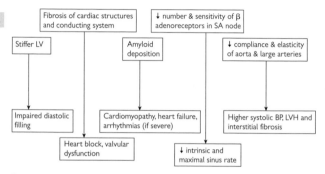

Fig. 1.2 Changes in cardiovascular system with healthy ageing. SA, sinoatrial; LV, left ventricular; BP, blood pressure; LVH, left ventricular hypertrophy. (Adapted with permission from Stott D, Singh A (2006) Chapter 44, Cardiac Aging and Systemic Disorders. In: Pathy J, Sinclair AJ, Morley JE (eds) *Principles and Practice of geriatric medicine*. 4th ed. Chichester: WileyBlackwell).

Pharmacology and therapeutics in the elderly

The elderly consume about a third of all prescription medications, despite only accounting for 16% of the population. They are more likely to experience adverse drug reactions, which can result in serious consequences, and also to be taking multiple drugs with potential interactions. Despite the increased risks of pharmacological therapy in older patients, the elderly are not well represented in clinical trials and although this is improving (see Chapter 11) there is still a lot to be learned.

Adverse drug reactions

Some drugs are more likely to produce adverse effects in older people than in younger individuals. There is evidence to support this for the examples listed in Table 1.1.

Table 1.1 Adverse effects of drugs classes in the elderly

Drug class	Adverse effect
Diuretics	Dehydration, hyponatraemia, orthostatic hypotension, gout
Lidocaine	Confusion
Opiate analgesia	Confusion, constipation
Aspirin	Peptic ulcer disease, bleeding risk increased
Angiotensin-converting enzyme (ACE) inhibitors and angiotensin-receptor antagonists	Renal impairment, postural hypotension
Digoxin	Bradycardia, increased risk of toxicity due to reduced renal clearance
β-blockers	Symptomatic bradycardia and hypotension
Warfarin	Increased bleeding risk
Clopidogrel	Increased bleeding risk especially in combination with aspirin

Pharmacokinetics and pharmacodynamics

Pharmacokinetics comprises a number of factors – drug absorption, distribution, metabolism, and excretion. Pharmacodynamics involves the nature and effects of a drug in the body. An older person may be more responsive to a drug either due to altered pharmacokinetics (i.e. how much active component is available) or altered pharmacodynamics (i.e. the end-organ response). Some common examples of these alterations are illustrated in Table 1.2.

Table 1.2 Common examples of altered pharmacokinetics and pharmacodynamics in the elderly

Drug	Effect
Nifedipine, verapamil	High first pass effect, more likely to have greater bioavailability in the elderly due to reduced gut-associated cytochrome P450 activity
Digoxin	Higher doses may accumulate in older people due to reduced renal clearance
ACE inhibitors	Renal elimination impaired with advancing age
Furosemide	Older people less sensitive to diuretic effects
Warfarin	Older patients require lower doses to achieve anticoagulation than younger patients due to increase sensitivity
Propanolol and β blockers	Older patients more sensitive to β_1 effects leading to more marked reduction in heart rate
Amlodipine, enalapril, nifedipine, verapamil	Hepatic metabolism impaired with advancing age

Compliance

Effective pharmacotherapy relies on concordance with a prescribed medication regimen. Unfortunately, there is a lot of evidence than non-compliance with medication is common in the elderly population, although this is thought to be due to the number of medications and the duration of therapy, rather than an effect isolated to the elderly population. There are a number of factors involved:

- Number of medications
- Size of tablets – larger tablets more difficult to swallow, smaller ones more difficult to manipulate if dexterity reduced
- Cognitive impairment
- Unwanted side effects – e.g. urinary urgency secondary to diuretics in a patient with overactive bladder
- Visual impairment – difficulty reading or distinguishing between medications
- Drug-disease interactions – a number of sets of criteria have been formulated to help guide prescription of medication in the elderly

Beers criteria is a list of medication that should be avoided or used with great caution in the elderly. It is published in the USA.

STOPP (Screening Tool of Older Persons Prescriptions) comprises 65 clinically significant criteria for potentially inappropriate prescribing in older people.

START (Screening Tool to Alert doctors to Right Treatment) consists of 22 evidence-based prescribing indicators for commonly encountered diseases in older people.

Hints and tips for prescribing in the elderly

- Start low and go slow – that is, start any new medications at a low dose and monitor for unwanted effects before increasing in small increments.
- Review the entire medication regimen before starting any new medication.
- Consider the use of non-pharmacological therapy if appropriate.
- Consider the risks and benefits of any new medication.
- Perform regular medication reviews and withdraw drugs that are inappropriate or no longer necessary.

Improving concordance in the elderly

Concordance involves prescribing with rather than for patients with the aim of improving compliance and reducing drug wastage (non-use). It is often perceived as difficult to put into practice especially in the elderly. Barriers include motivation, healthcare beliefs, cultural beliefs, and cognitive decline.

The key to improving concordance is patient and carer education so that they understand the reason for and the benefits of treatment in both the short and longer term. Even in the frail elderly, self-management should be encouraged. As healthcare professions it is our responsibility to spend the necessary time educating our patients, irrespective of age.

Involvement of specialist nurses, pharmacists, and community matrons is key to helping patients' understanding of their disease and the need for treatment, as well as facilitating self-management. This has been shown to be effective in both diabetes and heart failure, two common problems in the elderly.

Cardiac rehabilitation programmes are beneficial in improving concordance, but the elderly are often excluded due to physical disabilities, limited availability and access, lack of awareness of benefit or self-refusal. Attendance should be encouraged and facilitated by having more user-friendly facilities that older people can and will attend.

Educational material should be user-friendly and take into account sensory and physical impairments associated with age (especially visual and hearing impairment).

Impacts of co-morbidities in the elderly

Cardiac disease is common and therefore so is the incidence of cardiac dysfunction with non-cardiac disease. Non-cardiac disease may be secondary to cardiac disease, or may be unrelated. Similarly, as there is reduced cardiac homeostatic reserve, the elderly are more susceptible to cardiac manifestations of non-cardiac disease (see Table 1.3).

Table 1.3 Impacts of co-morbidities in the elderly

Organ/system	Secondary effects of cardiac disease (or treatment of) on organ	Secondary effects of organ disease on heart
Brain	Acute stroke secondary to arrhythmias (e.g. AF), hypertension, embolism	Neurological defects may lead to reduced mobility and less benefit from rehabilitation and exercise
	CCF and AF associated with cognitive decline and dementia	Cognitive impairment may affect medication compliance
Lungs	Pulmonary hypertension	Right heart failure, CCF and AF common complications of chronic respiratory disease
		Respiratory infections result in increased risk of hospitalization for heart failure (increased cytokines associated with negative inotropic effects is one postulated mechanism)
Gastrointestinal	Aspirin can cause acute/chronic gastrointestinal haemorrhage	Acute gastrointestinal haemorrhage more likely to result in circulatory collapse due to reduced homeostatic reserve
	Association between aortic stenosis and angiodysplasia	Chronic gastrointestinal blood loss may exacerbate symptoms of ischaemic heart disease due to anaemia
Renal	Reduced cardiac output results in renal hypoperfusion and decline in renal function	Renal impairment associated with increased risk of cardiovascular disease
Endocrine	Diabetic patients at high risk of ischaemic heart disease and CCF. May present atypically (e.g. silent myocardial infarction)	Hyperthyroidism causes arrhythmias (e.g. AF), palpitations, and hypertension
		Hypothyroidism causes bradycardia, pericardial effusion, CCF, and hypertension
	Thyroid replacement therapy may cause myocardial infarction or exacerbate ischaemic heart disease	Acromegaly associated with hypertension and cardiomyopathy

Table 1.3 (*Contd.*)

Organ/system	Secondary effects of cardiac disease (or treatment of) on organ	Secondary effects of organ disease on heart
Infections	Patients with CCF more at risk of infections	Chronic sepsis and increased invasive therapy in the elderly associated with risk of infective endocarditis
Nutrition	Cachexia secondary to CCF associated with higher mortality than CCF alone	Low body mass index associated with higher complication rate post-cardiac surgery

CCF, congestive heart failure; AF, atrial fibrillation.

References and recommended reading

Bracewell C, Gray R, Rai GS (2010) *Essential facts in geriatric medicine*. Oxford: Radcliffe.

Department of Health (2001) *National service framework for older people. Medicines and older people*. London: Department of Health.

Evans G, Williams F (2000) *Oxford textbook of geriatric medicine*. 2nd edn. Oxford: Oxford University Press.

Fick DM, Cooper JW, Wade WE, Waller JL, Maclean JR, Beers MH (2003) Medications to be avoided or used with caution in older patients. Updating the Beers criteria for potentially inappropriate medication use in older adults: results of a US consensus panel of experts. *Arch Intern Med* **163**:2716–24.

Gallagher P, Ryan C, Byrne S, Kennedy J, O'Mahony D (2008) STOPP (Screening Tool of Older Persons Prescriptions) and START (Screening Tool to Alert doctors to Right Treatment). Consensus validation. *Int J Clin Pharmacol Ther* **46**:72–83.

National Statistics Online – http://www.nationalstatisticsoffice.gov.uk.

Royal College of Physicians (1997) *Medication for older people*. 2nd edn. London, Royal College of Physicians.

Stott D, Singh A (2006) Chapter 44, Cardiac Aging and Systemic Disorders. In: Pathy J, Sinclair AJ, Morley JE. (eds) *Principles and practice of geriatric medicine*. 4th edn. Chichester: John Wiley.

Chapter 2

Ischaemic heart disease in the elderly

Introduction

- Incidence and prevalence of ischaemic heart disease (IHD) rise greatly with age: >30% people aged >65 years in the developed world have angina or myocardial infarction (MI) and a further 30% have covert (asymptomatic) disease.
- The prevalence is similar in males and females in elderly population.
- Most common cause of death in the elderly.
- There is a high proportion of elderly patients (>30% are >75 years) in registries but they only represent 10% of those included in clinical trials. The patients in clinical trials generally have less co-morbid disease so there is lack of a good evidence base for treatment. Where there is evidence we know that elderly patients do benefit even from invasive strategies, albeit at a greater procedural and bleeding risk. Thus age alone should not be a contraindication to treatment.

Presentation

- Symptoms may be vague or non-specific, e.g. confusion, fall, lethargy.
- Pulmonary oedema may be the first manifestation of IHD in older people; indeed older people with severe coronary artery disease may experience recurrent pulmonary oedema but have normal systolic function on echo. This can result from an episode of ischaemia, causing elevation of left atrial pressure secondary to impaired diastolic filling.
- Other important causes of chest pain and shortness of breath that should be considered in the acute setting include
  - Pneumonia
  - Acute exacerbation of chronic obstructive lung disease (COPD)
  - Asthma
  - Pulmonory embolism
  - Aortic dissection
  - Cardiac tamponode
  - Pericarditis
  - Oesophasitis/peptic ulcer.

History	Shortness of breath on exertion
	Chest pain
	Shoulder/back/neck/abdominal pain
	Dizziness
	Nausea
	Perspiration
	Collapse
	Risk factors (see p. 22)
Examination	May be normal, even if patient has severe coronary artery disease
	Fourth heart sound may indicate impaired diastolic function
	Apex beat sustained if cardiac hypertrophy present
	Look for evidence of anaemia or thyroid over/underactivity – may be the underlying cause of new onset angina symptoms
	Palpate peripheral pulses (i.e. look for evidence of vascular disease)
	Auscultate for renal and carotid bruits (i.e. look for evidence of vascular disease)

Diagnostic issues in the elderly

- Ageing is associated with impaired perception of ischaemic cardiac pain; myocardial ischaemia may be 'silent', i.e. asymptomatic.
- Shortness of breath on exertion is more common than chest pain as a clinical manifestation of IHD.
- Other co-morbidities may limit exertion, hence angina symptoms may be related to different circumstances, e.g. cold weather, anxiety, post prandial.
- The character of angina pain in elderly people may be atypical, e.g. burning, epigastric pain, or pain in the back or shoulders alone. These may be misdiagnosed as peptic ulcer disease or osteoarthritic pain.
- Investigation of angina may be limited by co-morbidities, e.g. patients with musculoskeletal, vascular, or neurological pathology may be unable to walk on the treadmill or use an exercise bike for the exercise stress test. Similarly, physical deconditioning may lead to early termination of exercise testing before a conclusive result can be obtained.
- ST segment depression and non-specific electrocardiographic (ECG) changes are more common than ST segment elevation in elderly patients with acute MI.
- Table 2.1 summarizes the key features of investigations recommended in ischaemic heart disease in the elderly.

Table 2.1 Investigation of ischaemic heart disease

Test	Indications	Positive/ high-risk result	Other
ECG	All patients	ST elevation	Often abnormal in older patients, e.g. resting ST depression, conduction defects
		New LBBB	
		ST depression	
			If ongoing symptoms, perform serial ECGs
			Pathological Q waves suggest previous MI
Cardiac biomarkers, e.g. troponin I, troponin T, CK-MB	Acute coronary syndrome	Varies according to assay	Venous sample should be taken 12 hours after chest pain peaks in severity
		Elevated troponin indicates increased risk in acute coronary syndrome and heart failure	Troponin may be elevated due to other co-morbidities and should be interpreted accordingly (see Other causes of elevated troponin T or I, p. 21)
			Troponin levels may remain elevated up to two weeks post-myocardial damage

Table 2.1 (*Contd.*)

Test	Indications	Positive/ high-risk result	Other
Chest X-ray	Acute coronary syndrome	Evidence of heart failure	
Exercise stress test	Patients with intermediate or high pre-test probability of coronary artery disease who are functionally able to manage walking on a treadmill or use an exercise bike	Early onset angina symptoms, >2 mm ST depression, low exercise tolerance or failure to increase systolic blood pressure	Interpretation includes symptomatic response, exercise capacity, haemodynamic response, and ECG response
Stress myocardial perfusion imaging	Baseline ECG shows LBBB, ST depression >1 mm, paced rhythm or pre-excitation (i.e. factors that would make interpretation on exercise ECG difficult) Poor exercise tolerance due to other co-morbidities Inconclusive exercise test Preoperative assessment (see Chapter 12)	Large anterior inducible defects, multiple moderate-sized inducible defects, left ventricular dilatation or left ventricular dysfunction Can detect viable myocardium and help predict benefit of revascularization in some patients	Either exercise stress or pharmacological vasodilator stress (dipyridamole, adenosine or dobutamine) (see Fig. 2.1)
Stress echo	Baseline ECG shows LBBB, ST depression >1 mm, paced rhythm or pre-excitation (i.e. factors that would make interpretation on exercise ECG difficult)	As above – preferred test largely depends on local availability and expertise	Dobutamine is usual agent used
Echo (resting)	Aortic outflow murmur Heart failure Pulmonary oedema	Regional wall motion abnormality	May detect previous MI (regional wall motion abnormality), diastolic dysfunction (prolongation of flow through mitral valve) in addition to valve abnormalities

(*Contd.*)

Table 2.1 (*Contd.*)

Test	Indications	Positive/ high-risk result	Other
Coronary angiography	Persistent angina despite optimal medical management	Significant coronary artery stenosis (>50%)	More difficult in older patients due to tortuous, calcified iliofemoral vessels and atheromatous aorta
	Patients identified as 'high risk' by non-invasive testing (e.g. exercise stress test or stress imaging), high pre-test probability of coronary artery disease (e.g. TIMI score p. 28)		Should be considered early in patients with acute coronary syndrome
			Contraindications include sepsis, recent neurological event, renal failure, allergy to contrast media

ECG, electrocardiogram; LBBB, left bundle branch block; MI, myocardial infarction; CK-MB, creatine kinase MB

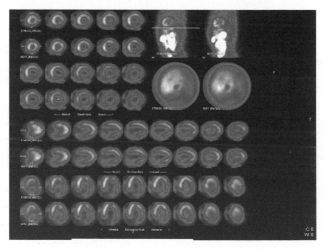

Fig. 2.1 Stress myocardial perfusion image showing evidence of full thickness infarction in the basal inferior wall and partial thickness infarction throughout the remaining inferior wall with mild inducible ischaemia in the lateral wall only; evidence of impaired left ventricular function with ejection fraction 35%.

Other causes of elevated troponin T or I

Troponin T or I levels may be raised in:

- Sepsis
- Hypovolaemia
- Atrial fibrillation
- Congestive cardiac failure
- Myocarditis
- Myocardial contusion
- Pulmonary embolus and pulmonary hypertension
- Renal failure – acute or chronic
- Respiratory failure
- Rhabdomyolysis
- Aortic dissection
- Acute stroke and subarachnoid haemorrhage
- Apical ballooning syndrome.

Risk factors

Smoking

Cigarette smoking at least doubles the risk of new coronary events in elderly people, and elderly patients who smoke should be encouraged and supported to stop smoking. Stopping smoking at an older age is still associated with survival improvements.

Hypertension

Approximately two-thirds of elderly hypertensive patients have isolated systolic hypertension (systolic blood pressure (BP) ≥140 mmHg, diastolic BP ≤90 mmHg). There is now good evidence that treatment of hypertension reduces cardiovascular mortality; management of hypertension is addressed in Chapter 9. While β-blockers are no longer regarded as first-line treatment in hypertension, they should be used in patients with IHD unless contraindicated.

Dyslipidaemia

High serum total cholesterol and low serum high-density lipoprotein (HDL) are risk factors for coronary events in the elderly. However, many patients with coronary artery disease have 'normal' total cholesterol levels. Statin therapy has been shown to reduce mortality and morbidity even in patients with normal cholesterol levels and should be prescribed to elderly patients with IHD unless contraindicated or if the patient has another life-threatening condition.

Diabetes mellitus

Elderly diabetic patients without known IHD are at higher risk of new coronary events than non-diabetic patients with IHD. They are also more likely to be hypertensive and have dyslipidaemia, which further increases their risk of cardiovascular events. Good blood pressure control is especially important in reducing cardiovascular events in diabetic patients. Diabetic control is also important and should be optimized. Treatment options are dietary modification and appropriate medication (e.g. metformin ± sulphonylurea ± insulin) to maintain HbA_1C <6.5%. This target may need to be modified in the elderly patient if the risk of hypoglycaemia is considered high. Metformin appears to be superior to other therapies in terms of reducing cardiovascular mortality, so it should be prescribed as first-line if tolerated and the glomerular filtration rate (GFR) is ≥45 ml (see the National Institute for Health and Clinical Excellence (NICE) guidelines on type 2 diabetes (NICE 2008)). Thiazolidinediones should be avoided if possible because of risk of precipitating heart failure and recent evidence suggesting increased risk of cardiovascular events and fractures. Other new agents such as gliptins and exenatide are available and should be used in consultation with a diabetologist (see the NICE guidelines on newer agents for type 2 diabetes (NICE 2009)).

Obesity

Obesity is an independent risk factor for new IHD events and should be managed with weight reduction (dietary modification and aerobic exercise). This should be encouraged even in the elderly and has additional health benefits. There is a need to develop more accessible diet and exercise programmes (see below) specifically for the elderly obese patient.

Physical inactivity

Physical inactivity is associated with hypertension, dyslipidaemia, and obesity, thus increasing the risk of cardiovascular morbidity and mortality. Examples of exercise programmes suitable for the elderly are walking, climbing stairs, swimming, cycling, dancing, and tai chi. Some local gyms and day centres also offer supervised exercise sessions; these need to be developed and the elderly encouraged to attend.

Management of stable angina

Acute attack

In the event of an angina attack, the patient should be advised to:
- Stop any exertion and sit down
- Use glyceryl trinitrate (GTN) sublingually. Note: Elderly people are more susceptible vasodilation leading to symptomatic hypotension or headache and should be warned about this and given advice on what to do
- Repeat GTN administration if symptoms have not improved after 5 minutes
- If symptoms fail to improve after second dose of GTN, call 999.

When reviewing patients with IHD, always check the expiry date on their GTN preparations as oral preparations deteriorate rapidly (months).

Medical management of stable angina

All patients should be treated with aspirin 75 mg od, unless contraindicated. In those with aspirin allergy, clopidogrel 75 mg is the current recommended alternative. Patients with peptic ulcer disease should be prescribed aspirin and a proton pump inhibitor (PPI). Clopidogrel is an alternative, but avoid co-prescription of clopidogrel and PPI as there is some evidence but at present not conclusive that this may reduce antiplatelet efficacy (we advise prescribing ranitidine as an alternative until more data are available.)

Cardiovascular risk factors (see Risk factors, p. 22) should also be addressed. Anti-anginal medication is less well tolerated in older people and all agents have potential side effects.

If a patient has symptoms infrequently (<1 per week), treat with GTN prn, aspirin and a β-blocker if this is tolerated. If the patient experiences symptoms more frequently, they may benefit from one of the prophylactic oral medications listed in Table 2.2.

Table 2.2 Prophylactic oral medications for stable angina

Drug	Mode of action	Side effects	Notes
β-Blockers, e.g. atenolol, bisoprolol, metoprolol	Inhibition of cardiac β receptors causing reduced heart rate and cardiac work	May exacerbate claudication May mask symptoms of hypoglycaemia, i.e. use with caution in diabetic patients on hypoglycaemic agents Bradycardia Cold extremities Fatigue Hypotension and postural hypotension	Recommended as first-line therapy if tolerated Caution if hypotension, postural hypotension or first-degree heart block Contraindicated in patients with history of reversible airway obstruction (e.g. asthma, COPD with reversibility), bradycardia, sick sinus syndrome, high degree AV block, decompensated LV failure
Ca²⁺ channel blockers: two types Dihydropyridine, e.g. amlodipine Non-dihydropyridine (rate slowing), e.g. verapamil, diltiazem	Peripheral arteriolar dilation, reduction in afterload → reduced cardiac work	Peripheral oedema Bradycardia Hypotension Postural hypotension	Useful alternative first-line therapy in patients intolerant of β-blockers Avoid concurrent use of verapamil/diltiazem and β-blockers due to additive effects on heart rate Use with caution if heart failure as negatively inotropic Monitor for postural hypotension
Long acting nitrates, e.g. isosorbide mononitrate	Peripheral vasodilatation → reduction in end-diastolic ventricular volume, reduction of distension of heart wall → reduction of oxygen demand	Headaches Hypotension Reflex tachycardia	Ensure patient has nitrate-free period of at least 8 hours per day, to avoid developing tolerance Also available as patch preparation
Nicorandil	Coronary vasodilator	Hypotension Headache Flushing	Tolerance may develop

COPD, chronic obstructive pulmonary disease; AV, atrioventricular; LV, left ventricular.

Coronary revascularization

Patients with persistent angina despite medical therapy may be considered for coronary revascularization. Coronary revascularization can be performed either percutaneously (see Percutaneous coronary intervention in elderly patients, p. 36) or via coronary artery bypass surgery (see Surgery for ischaemic heart disease, p. 38).

Revascularization in the elderly – current evidence

Unfortunately the elderly are poorly represented even in recent trials with the exception of the TIME and APPROACH trials discussed in Chapter 11. These trails confirmed that revascularization with coronary artery bypass graft (CABG) or percutaneous coronary intervention (PCI) was beneficial in elderly patients (>70 years) with evidence of improved survival and quality of life. The COURAGE trial published in 2007 compared optimal medical therapy versus PCI plus optimal medical therapy in 2287 patients with stable angina. The study found no difference between the groups in the primary endpoint of death or MI. There was an early benefit of PCI on symptoms, functional ability, and quality of life at six months but this was lost by 36 months. The average age was 62 ± 10 and 85% of the sample was male, so the sample was not representative of the elderly population. The implications of this are that PCI should be performed for limiting symptoms in patients with stable angina but optimal medical therapy is a safe and viable alternative. CABG is associated with significant mortality benefits and symptom improvement at five years but unfortunately there are no good trials in the elderly comparing this procedure with optimal medical management. The debate on CABG versus PCI continues but the SYNTAX trial (1800 patients; mean age 65 ± 9.8, >75% male) published in 2009 showed that CABG was superior to PCI with drug-eluting stents in patients with three-vessel disease or left main stem disease with a lower rate of major adverse cardiac or cerebrovascular events at 1 year. Therefore CABG should be considered in the elderly patient with suitable anatomical disease if indicated for symptoms, but many patients may opt for the less invasive PCI and accept a higher revascularization rate.

Management of acute coronary syndromes

Management of acute coronary syndromes is based on current evidence. New NICE guidelines for NSTEMI and unstable angina were published in March 2010 (www.nice.org.uk/CG94).

Acute coronary syndrome is divided into three clinical categories:

1. ST elevation MI (STEMI)
- >2 mm ST elevation in ≥2 adjacent chest leads (Fig. 2.2) or >1 mm ST elevation in ≥2 other leads or new left bundle branch block (LBBB).
- If there is inferior STEMI (ST elevation in II, III, aVF), perform right-sided ECG to look for right ventricular infarction.

2. Non-ST elevation MI (NSTEMI)
- ECG does not show ST elevation but troponin level is elevated.
- ECG may show ST depression or new T inversion but may be normal (Fig. 2.3).

3. Unstable angina
- History of angina symptoms at rest, new onset and severe angina, crescendo angina or post MI.
- Non-specific ECG changes (e.g. ST depression, T inversion) but troponin not elevated.

The TIMI score has been widely used to identify patients at high risk of mortality and predict need for early revascularization (see Box 2.2). The recent NICE guidelines recommend the GRACE score (Global Registry of Acute Coronary Events) to assess the risk of future adverse cardiovascular events. The score is weighted and is available online at www.outcomes-umassmed.org/grace/. The factors to include are shown in Box 2.1. Patients are defined as low, intermediate or high risk.

Box 2.1 Factors to include when assessing risk with GRACE scoring system

Full history (age, previous MI, Previous PCI or CABG)
Physical examination (pulse and BP and evidence of heart failure)
ECG
Blood tests (troponin, creatinine, FBC and glucose)

MI, myocardial infarction; PCI, percutaneous coronary intervention; CABG, coronary artery bypass grafting; BP, blood pressure; ECG, electrocardiogram; FBC, full blood count

Box 2.2 TIMI scoring system

	TIMI score	
Age >65 years	1	0–2 Low risk
≥3 cardiovascular risk factors	1	3–4 Intermediate risk
ST changes on ECG	1	5–7 High risk
Elevated troponin	1	
Previous coronary stenosis	1	
>2 episodes angina in preceding 24 hours	1	
Use of aspirin in previous 1 week	1	

Acute management

Aims are to relieve pain and distress and to treat life-threatening instability. For **all** patients, give:

- High-flow oxygen (but not if known COPD)
- 300 mg aspirin po – reduces incidence of death and non-fatal MI in patients with unstable angina
- Clopidogrel 300–600 mg po (if >75 years give 300 mg due to increased bleeding risk)
- Morphine intravenously with anti-emetic for pain relief
- If admission glucose ≥ 10mmol start insulin sliding scale
- GTN ± intravenous (iv) morphine (+ antiemetic) for analgesia
- If symptoms persist, iv GTN infusion.

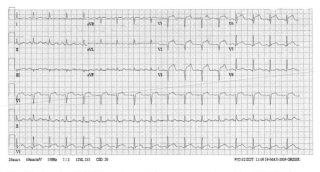

Fig. 2.2 Anterior STEMI in a 78-year-old woman presenting with one hour of central chest pain. Primary percutaneous coronary intervention with a drug-eluting stent was performed on admission. The patient made a good recovery and was discharged two days later; she remains well and angina-free 12 months post procedure.

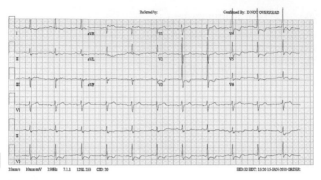

Fig. 2.3 ECG of a 75-year-old man presenting with dyspnoea. There is anterolateral ischaemia and troponin was 1.2 Ng/ml. Patient had angiography during admission and a drug-eluting stent was inserted into the left anterior descending artery.

Patients with STEMI

For patients with STEMI, treat with aspirin, clopidogrel, oxygen, and analgesia, plus:

- Aim for prompt revascularization with PCI within 90 minutes of presentation. This is the preferred treatment strategy for most elderly patients unless there are contraindications (see Box 2.1).
- If PCI is not available, aim for thrombolysis within 30 minutes of presentation (if <12 hours since onset of symptoms). At present guidelines recommend recombinant tissue plasminogen activator (rtPA) (alteplase, reteplase, or tenecteplase). The risk of major bleeding, both cerebral and non-cerebral is increased in the elderly (>75), in females, those with low body mass index, and systolic and diastolic hypertension, so PCI is preferable in these patients if it is available.
- After thrombolysis, early angiography should be performed (if there are no contraindications) to determine the most appropriate reperfusion strategy (see pp. 36–39).
- Low molecular weight heparin subcutaneously (sc) (e.g. enoxaparin) or fondaparinux.
- Commence β-blocker unless contraindicated.
- Monitor closely (telemetry) for arrhythmias and heart failure.

Box 2.3 Contraindications to thrombolysis

Absolute contraindications to thrombolysis	Prior intracranial haemorrhage
	Known malignant intracranial lesion or arteriovenous malformation
	Ischaemic stroke in preceding 3 months
	Suspected aortic dissection
	Active bleeding or bleeding diathesis
	Significant closed head or facial trauma in preceding 3 months
	Surgical procedure in preceding 1 month
Relative contraindications to thrombolysis	Uncontrolled hypertension (>200/120), if fails to reduce after analgesia and B-blocker ± nitrates
	Severe diabetic retinopathy with untreated neovascularization
	Peptic ulceration – currently symptomatic

Patients with NSTEMI

For patients with NSTEMI, treat with aspirin, oxygen, and analgesia, plus:
- Clopidogrel 300 mg loading dose then 75 mg od thereafter.
Note: Do not give clopidogrel if urgent (<1/52) CABG is anticipated
- Low molecular weight heparin sc (e.g. enoxaparin). Fondaparinux sc is recommended in patients without high bleeding risk (Box 2.4) unless urgent angiography planned (within 24 hours)
- Risk assessment using GRACE or TIMI (see p. 28)
- Commence β-blocker unless contraindicated
- Monitor closely (telemetry) for arrhythmias

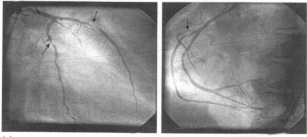

(a)   (b)

Fig. 2.1a, b Coronary angiography in a 74-year-old man with severe limiting angina and impaired left ventricular function. There is severe proximal disease in all three vessels as indicated by arrows. The patient had a coronary artery bypass graft and is angina-free with good exercise tolerance two years post surgery.

- Consider early coronary angiography ± revascularization if intermediate or high risk on GRACE or TIMI and no contraindication. Invasive approach may not be appropriate for all patients, e.g. those with serious co-morbidities or other life-threatening conditions (Fig. 2.4).

Patients with unstable angina

For patients with unstable angina, treat with aspirin, oxygen, and analgesia, plus:

- Clopidogrel 300 mg loading dose then 75 mg od.
- Low molecular weight heparin sc (e.g. enoxaparin) or fondaparinux
- Commence β-blocker unless contraindicated
- Monitor closely (telemetry) for arrhythmias
- Consider stress imaging once patient stable (Table 2.1, p. 18)
- Consider coronary angiography ± revascularization if symptoms fail to respond to medical therapy or high risk on GRACE or TIMI score (p. 28). An invasive approach may not be appropriate for all patients, e.g. those with serious co-morbidities or other life-threatening conditions.

Other antiplatelet therapies to consider

- Prasugrel is a new and more potent thienopyridine than clopidogrel. NICE recently issued recommendations for its use in combination with aspirin in patients undergoing primary PCI for STEMI, patients who develop stent thrombosis while on clopidogrel treatment and in patients with diabetes mellitus and acute coronary syndrome undergoing PCI. Because of the high risk of major bleeding it should be avoided in patients >75 years of age or <60 kg in weight, and in those with active bleeding or history of transient ischaemic attack or stroke.
- Ticagrelor is a new class of antiplatelet agent that is orally active and binds the P2Y12 receptor. Early results are promising but it has not yet been approved for use in the UK.
- Three GPIIb/IIIa inhibitors have been approved for clinical use, namely abciximab, eptifibatide, and tirofiban. They are only available for iv use and there is limited evidence, especially in the elderly. They are considered in very high-risk patients and as an adjunct to PCI and should only be used on specialist advice. The risk of bleeding is high so they should be used with great caution in those >75 years.

Longer-term management (i.e. after first 24 hrs)

- Address risk factors, e.g. smoking cessation.
- Prescribe statin therapy if life expectancy >2 years.
- Continue aspirin 75 mg od (add a PPI if there is high risk of peptic ulceration, however, avoid PPIs in patients taking clopidogrel because of potential interaction and increased risk of cardiac events; use an alternative such as ranitidine). This is based on current recommendations and is likely to change.
- Continue dual antiplatelet therapy (DAT) with aspirin 75 mg and clopidogrel 75 mg for 3 months after STEMI and 12 months after NSTEMI. If a drug-eluting stent is inserted after STEMI, DAT is continued for 12 months.
- Continue with β-blockers if tolerated.
- Add an angiotensin-converting enzyme (ACE) inhibitor if tolerated. Angiotensin II receptor antagonists are an alternative if ACE inhibitors are not tolerated due to cough.
- Prescribe an aldosterone antagonist (eplerenone 25 mg od) if clinical heart failure or echo evidence of left ventricular dysfunction (ejection fraction <40%).
- Cardiac rehabilitation (see p. 40).
- Driving advice (see Driver and Vehicle Licensing Agency (DVLA) guidance at www.dft.gov.uk).
- Echocardiogram to assess left ventricular function. Asymptomatic left ventricular dysfunction is not uncommon in patients with IHD, especially in elderly patients; these patients should be treated with ACE inhibitors if tolerated (see Chapter 5).

Prognosis

Overall 10% patients die or have a further MI in hospital after an acute coronary syndrome, but in octogenarians this figure is almost doubled.

Box 2.4 Factors associated with high bleeding risk

Advancing age (especially > 85 yrs)
Known bleeding disorders
Renal impairment
Low body weight (< 60kg)

Complications of STEMI and NSTEMI

For detailed management of complications of STEMI and NSTEMI see Oxford Handbook of Cardiology, Chapter 4.

Short term	Long term
Cardiac	
Cardiac arrhythmias, e.g. bradycardia, complete heart block (inferior MI), first or second degree heart block, atrial fibrillation, ventricular arrhythmias	Further cardiac events (ischaemia/ infarction)
Cardiogenic shock	Congestive heart failure
Right heart failure secondary to right ventricular (RV) infarction	Stent thrombosis
Ventricular rupture, acute pericardial tamponade	
Ventricular aneurysm	Ventricular arrhythmias
Acute mitral regurgitation	
Post infarction pericarditis	
Acute pericardial tamponade	
Ventricular septal defect	
Other	
Depression	Depression
Stroke – intracranial haemorrhage or infarct	Loss of independence
Delirium	Loss of confidence
	Thrombocytopenia

Other issues post STEMI and NSTEMI in the elderly

- As discussed in Chapter 5, the benefit of intracardiac defibrillators in the elderly is still unclear but they should be considered in those who meet NICE guidelines and are expected to survive >12 months with a reasonable quality of life (see Chapter 5 for a summary of guidelines). Similarly for resynchronization therapy, see Chapter 5.
- DAT with aspirin and clopidogrel is associated with increased bleeding risk and this should be taken into account when deciding on whether to pursue an invasive strategy and the type of stent to be deployed (see Percutaneous coronary intervention in elderly patients, p. 36). Factors that increase bleeding risk include age, renal impairment, known gastrointestinal lesions, liver disease and thrombocytopenia. If elderly patients present with bleeding on DAT, treatment should be discontinued and the bleeding stopped as soon as possible. Unfortunately there are no suitable alternatives or antidotes. Remember transfusion may increase coagulability so avoid this unless the patient is compromised.

- The combination of DAT and anticoagulation with warfarin is sometimes necessary when warfarin is indicated for another reason, e.g. DVT or pulmonary embolism. This is associated with a high bleeding risk and should be avoided where possible, especially in those >75 years. If it is deemed essential it should be for as short a time as possible and close monitoring is essential.
- As discussed in Chapter 1, the elderly are at increased risk of complications from pharmacological therapy and this needs to be considered when planning long-term treatments. Elderly patients should not be denied treatments that are beneficial but there should be a greater emphasis on quality of life.

Percutaneous coronary intervention (PCI) in elderly patients

- Balloon angioplasty ± stent insertion. There are two main types of stent – bare metal and drug eluting. The latter elute sirolimus or paclitaxel to reduce rate of stent endothelialization and stenosis, and there are guidelines on their use. Drug-eluting stents require DAT for at least 12 months due to increased risk of late stent thrombosis, and this should be taken into consideration in elderly patients who are at greater risk of bleeding complications.
- Indications:
  - STEMI and NSTEMI
  - Angina not controlled with medical therapy and coronary anatomy suitable for PCI.
- There is good evidence that older patients benefit from PCI to the same degree as younger patients (i.e. primary success rate 70–90%). One-year post-PCI mortality is also lower than in patients treated with medical therapy alone. However, patients undergoing PCI are exposed to a procedural mortality risk of about 8%, related to major complications (e.g. MI, stroke, emergency coronary surgery, renal failure). They are also at risk of local vascular complications (e.g. severe haemorrhage, dissection, aneurysm formation, arterial occlusion). Quality of life 1 year post PCI is good in octogenarians in spite of high mortality, so age alone should not be a contraindication.

Surgery for ischaemic heart disease

- Elderly people have a higher incidence of left main stem disease, multi-vessel disease, poor left ventricular function, and concomitant valve disease. As a result, coronary artery surgery may be a better treatment option for some older patients than PCI or medical management.
- The mean age of patients undergoing cardiac surgery is increasing.
- Indications include symptoms that cannot be controlled with medication or PCI and diffuse disease (i.e. not appropriate for PCI).
- The operative mortality rate is higher than in younger patients, ranging from 4% (elective procedure) to 13% (emergency case). There is also a higher non-fatal complication rate (e.g. stroke, atrial fibrillation). This is due to a combination of more advanced coronary disease and higher rates of co-morbidities.
- Patients undergoing elective CABG should be screened for carotid artery disease as its presence increases the risk of perioperative stroke.
- Cognitive impairment is one of the major concerns of patients and carers post cardiac surgery. Better preoperative assessment of cognitive function (including the Mini-mental State Examination (MMSE) and if necessary psychological assessment) is essential as those with preoperative dysfunction are at greater risk.
- Factors that increase risk of morbidity and mortality post CABG:
  - Increasing New York Heart Association (NYHA) class or reduced LVEF
  - Increasing age
  - Recent MI or unstable angina
  - Reoperation
  - Reduced renal function
  - Cerebrovascular disease
  - COPD
  - Smoking history
  - Obesity
  - Diabetes mellitus.

Despite the higher early complication/mortality rate, CABG is generally well tolerated by the elderly and confers similar improvements in symptoms and quality of life as younger patients in carefully selected patients. In addition, the 5-year survival of patients who recover from surgery is, for example, 60–75% in octogenarians, comparable with an age/sex matched population. Advanced age alone should therefore not be a contraindication to CABG, if the longer-term benefits are felt to outweigh the procedural risk. It is important to involve the patient in their treatment decisions, taking into account the risks and benefits relevant to them, their functional capacity, and preferences.

Risk scores based on patient characteristics are available. In the risk scores Parsonnet and EuroSCORE (European system for cardiac operative risk evaluation), each risk factor is given a number of points which when added, provide an estimate of the percentage predicted mortality for a patient undergoing a particular procedure. They are both available online and are easy to use (www.mpoullis.com/Parsonnet.htm and www.euroscore.org). Their main drawback is poor prediction in high-risk subsets. EuroSCORE logistic (www.Euroscore.org/logistic/Euroscore.htm) is more suitable for risk prediction in high risk subjects. It uses the same risk factors with logistic regression rather than simple addition. Regardless of the system used, octogenarians invariably score high in terms of estimated risk of death on account of age and co-morbidity. This in turn may lead to difficulties in counselling as well as hesitation in offering and accepting surgery among elderly patients.

Cardiac rehabilitation

Cardiac rehabilitation is an integrated process of care, encompassing:

- *Exercise training* – aims to prevent the disability that may arise from acute coronary syndrome and improve quality of life. Exercise programmes are tailored to the individual, to ensure that they exercise at an appropriate intensity. The programmes have been found to improve exercise tolerance and functional capacity in elderly patients post MI but are underused.
- *Secondary prevention* – education, counselling, and behavioural strategies. Aims to reduce the risk of further cardiac events by optimizing pharmacological therapy (e.g. monitoring and encouraging concordance with medication) and health promotion (e.g. smoking cessation, dietary advice, increasing physical activity).
- *Psychosocial intervention* – aims to identify and treat patients who have anxiety and/or depression post cardiac event, in order to improve function and quality of life.

Indications

Indicated in all patients post cardiac event (including heart failure admission) who are able to mobilize and able to participate. Carers/family can also attend sessions to support the patient if they have cognitive impairment or sensory impairment. Home-based programmes are available in some areas and may be more acceptable to elderly patients, who traditionally are underrepresented in rehabilitation programmes.

Guidelines, references, and recommended reading

Aronow WS (2006) Chapter 46 Ischaemic Heart Disease in Elderly Persons. In: Pathy J, Sinclair AJ, Morley JE. *Principles and practice of geriatric medicine*. 4th edn. Chichester: John Wiley.

Boden WE, O'Rourke RA, Teo KK, et al. (2007) Optimal medical therapy with or without PCI for stable coronary disease. *N Engl J Med* **356**:1503–16.

Eagle K, Guyton R (2004) ACC/AHA 2004 Guideline update for coronary artery bypass surgery. American College of Cardiology Foundation and Heart Association Inc.

Evans G, Williams F (2000) *Oxford textbook of geriatric medicine*. 2nd edn. Oxford: Oxford University Press.

Guidelines for the diagnosis and treatment of non-ST-segment elevation acute coronary syndromes (2007) The Task Force for the diagnosis and treatment of non-ST-segment elevation acute coronary syndromes of the European Society of Cardiology. *Eur Heart J* **28**:1598–660. Available at: www.escardio.org/guidelines.

Management of acute myocardial infarction in patients presenting with persistent ST-segment elevation (2008) The Task Force on the management of ST-segment elevation acute myocardial infarction of the European Society of Cardiology. *Eur Heart J* **29**:2909–45. Available: at: www.escardio.org/guidelines.

National Institute for Health and Clinical Excellence (2006) Implantable cardioverter defibrillators (ICDs) for the treatment of arrhythmias (review of TA11). Technology appraisal guidance 95. London: National Institute for Health and Clinical Excellence. Available at: www.nice.org.uk/ta95.

National Institute for Health and Clinical Excellence (2007) Cardiac resynchronisation therapy for the treatment of heart failure. Technology appraisal 120. London: National Institute for Health and Clinical Excellence. Available at: www.nice.org.uk/ta120.

National Institute for Health and Clinical Excellence (2008) Type 2 diabetes: the management of type 2 diabetes (update) Clinical guideline 66. London: National Institute for Health and Clinical Excellence. Available at: www.nice.org.uk/cg66.

National Institute for Health and Clinical Excellence (2009) Type 2 diabetes – newer agents (partial update of CG66). Clinical guideline 87. London: National Institute for Health and Clinical Excellence. Available at: www.nice.org.uk/cg87.

National Institute for Health and Clinical Excellence (2009) Prasugrel for the treatment of acute coronary syndromes with percutaneous coronary intervention. Technology appraisal 182. London: National Institute for Health and Clinical Excellence. Available at: www.nice.org.uk/ta182.

National Institute for Health and Clinical Excellence (2009) Drug-eluting stents for the treatment of coronary artery disease. Technology appraisal 152. London: National Institute for Health and Clinical Excellence. Available at: www.nice.org.uk/ta152.

NICE Guidelines (2010) The early management of unstable angina and non-ST-elevation myocardial infarction. Clinical giudeline 94. Available at: www.nice.org.uk/cg94.

Ramrakha D, Mill J (2006) *Oxford Handbook of Cardiology*, Chapter 4 'Coronary Artery Disease'. www.oup.com/uk/medicine/handbooks.

Serruys P, Morice MC, Kappetein AP, et al. (2009) Percutaneous coronary intervention versus coronary-artery bypass grafting for severe coronary artery disease. *N Engl J Med* **360**:961–72.

Scottish Intercollegiate Guidelines Network (2007) Acute coronary syndromes. Guideline 93. Edinburgh: Scottish Intercollegiate Guidelines Network. Available at: www.sign.ac.uk/pdf/sign93.pdf.

Scottish Intercollegiate Guidelines Network (2007) Management of stable angina. Guideline 96. Edinburgh: Scottish Intercollegiate Guidelines Network. Available at: www.sign.ac.uk/pdf/sign96.pdf.

Chapter 3

Valve disease

Valve disease

This chapter will discuss:
- The presentation and management of common valve lesions in the elderly
- Valve surgery in the elderly.

Valvular heart disease is an important cause of morbidity and mortality in elderly people. The classic clinical picture of valve disease may be obscured by age-related cardiovascular changes, other cardiac disease, and the presence of non-cardiac pathology.

Aortic stenosis

- Calcific aortic stenosis (AS) is the commonest valve disorder in the elderly and accounts for two-thirds of valve surgery cases.
- In a population-based study, significant aortic stenosis was found in 2.9% of randomly selected people aged 75–86 years, half of whom were symptomatic.
- Patients with AS may remain asymptomatic for many years and the prognosis in the asymptomatic patient is relatively good (Figure 3.1). Once symptoms develop the prognosis is poor with death occurring in approximately 2 years.
- Calcification of normal valve tissue increases with age and a proportion of these valves progress to significant stenosis. The factors that determine this progression are unclear.
- An association between AS and idiopathic gastrointestinal bleeding, and more specifically, intestinal angiodysplasia is recognised in the elderly, but the nature of this association is unclear.

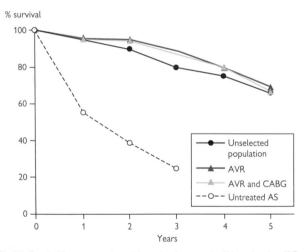

Fig. 3.1 Survival for octogenarians with aortic valve stenosis. AV, aortic valve; AVR, aortic valve replacement; CABG, coronary artery bypass graft. (Data adapted from Gehlot A, Mullany CJ, Ilstrup D, *et al.* (1996) Aortic valve replacement in patients aged 80 years and older: early and long-term results. *J Thorac Cardiovasc Surg* **111**:1026–36).

Symptoms and signs of AS in the elderly (Table 3.1)

• The main symptoms are angina pectoris, heart failure, and exertional syncope. Angina is often the initial symptom and associated coronary artery disease is found in about 50%. Calcific embolization with stroke, transient ischaemic attack (TIA), or other embolic event is a rare manifestation of AS.

• The clinical diagnosis of AS in the elderly may be difficult as the physical signs that indicate severity may be obscured by age-related vascular changes. An anacrotic pulse is uncommon and more likely to be felt in the left brachial or carotid. Hypertension may coexist with severe AS. Therefore, AS should be suspected in elderly patients with a characteristic harsh, long ejection systolic murmur, even in the absence of other physical signs.

Table 3.1 Clinical features of aortic valve disease

Aortic stenosis		Aortic regurgitation	
Symptoms	**Signs**	**Symptoms**	**Signs**
Asymptomatic	Anacrotic pulse*	Asymptomatic	Collapsing pulse
Angina pectoris	Low pulse pressure*		Wide pulse pressure
Heart failure	Ejection systolic murmur at base, aortic area, left sternal edge and carotids	Heart failure	Diastolic murmur at left sternal edge ± mid-diastolic
Dyspnoea		Dyspnoea	
Orthopnoea		Orthopnoea	Austin–Flint murmur
PND		PND	
Syncope	Left ventricular heave		Displaced apex beat
	Soft/inaudible S2*		

*May be absent in the elderly (see text for details). PND, paroxysmal nocturnal dyspnoea.

Investigations

Electrocardiogram (ECG): May show left ventricular hypertrophy (LVH) or left bundle branch block (LBBB) (see Fig. 3.2).

Chest radiograph (CXR) – may show aortic valve calcification and signs of congestion.

Doppler echocardiography – is currently the definitive technique and can define the severity of the stenosis (both transvalvular gradient and valve area) as well as left ventricular function and the presence of other valve lesions (Fig. 3.3).

Dobutamine stress echocardiography – in patients with low-flow (due to cardiac failure) low-gradient AS it can sometimes be difficult to differentiate between true severe AS and pseudo AS, where the valve is only mildly or moderately stenotic but the stenosis appears severe due to limitations in determining disease severity under low-flow conditions. Valve replacement is likely to benefit the former group, but may have little benefit in the latter. Dobutamine stress can distinguish 'true' and 'pseudo-severe' AS, and can evaluate contractile reserve, one of the strongest predictors of patient outcome from surgery.

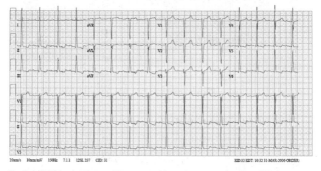

Fig. 3.2 ECG in an 84-year-old woman with aortic stenosis (gradient 82) showing first-degree heart block, left ventricular hypertrophy, and repolarization abnormality.

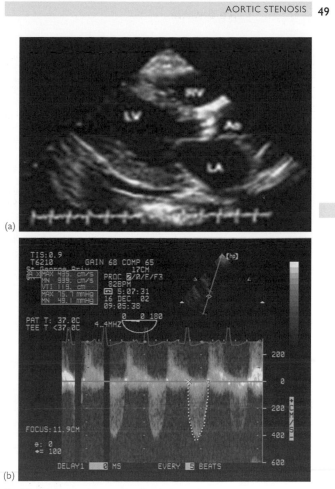

Fig. 3.3 Calcific aortic stenosis (a) with calculation of the transvalvular gradient using Doppler in (b). The peak gradient is 76 mmHg, indicating severe AS.

Management of AS

(See also Fig. 3.4.)

- In severe stenosis (transvalvular gradient >50 mmHg), patients <80 years, who are otherwise fit and active, should be referred for further assessment and consideration of valve replacement.
- In mild (gradient <30) or moderate stenosis (gradient 30–49), regular review is essential to determine progression and or the development of symptoms. Most cardiologists recommend annual echocardiograms as part of this assessment.
- Recently there has been interest in the use of statins and angiotensin-converting enzyme (ACE) inhibitors to delay the progression of AS based on the finding that patients with AS share many risk factors with atherosclerosis. However, as yet there is no conclusive evidence that use of either drug group is beneficial.

Indications for open valve replacement surgery in the elderly

Symptoms: Consider replacement of a stenotic aortic valve ± myocardial revascularization limited to major coronary arteries unless there are contraindications as follows:

- Consider valve replacement in asymptomatic patients <80 years with severe stenosis (see Management of AS, p. 50), good left ventricular function, and quality of life, in whom there is evidence that valve disease is progressing and likely to cause complications.
- Consider valve replacement for moderate stenosis (with a transvalvular gradient between 30 and 49 mmHg and a valve orifice area between 1 and 1.2 cm^2) in patients undergoing coronary revascularization, on the basis that the replacement only marginally increases the operative risk and progression of AS can be rapid, quickly negating the benefit of bypass surgery.

Type of valve: This requires careful consideration in each individual patient looking at risks and other indications for anticoagulation (e.g. atrial fibrillation). In most patients over 80 years, a tissue valve (bioprosthesis) that does not require anticoagulation is inserted as their life expectancy is shorter than the expected functional time of the biological prosthesis. One concern is in patients with a small annulus (<21 mm in diameter) as the high transvalvular gradient of tissue valves in these patients may limit offloading and haemodynamic benefit. Stentless bioprosthesis have lower gradients but are technically more difficult to insert; however, they will no doubt improve with advancing technology.

Outcome of surgery for AS

In selected elderly patients over 80 years, the postoperatively mortality from aortic valve replacement (AVR) is 5–10% (compared with 2–3% in younger patients). The addition of a coronary artery bypass graft (CABG) increases this to 15–20%. After successful surgery, survival is similar to a control population with rates of 95%, 80%, and 70% at one, three, and five years, respectively, and compared with 57%, 37%, and 25% at one, two, and three years, respectively, in those who decline surgery. Ninety per cent of patients return to their own homes and lead an independent life after successful surgery (Prêtre and Turina 2003).

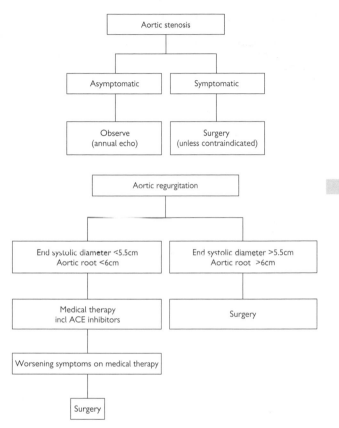

Fig. 3.4 Management of aortic valve disease. ACE, angiotensin-converting enzyme.

Transcatheter aortic valve replacement

- A self-expanding, tri-level frame, porcine pericardium heart valve has been developed that can be inserted percutaneously (transcatheter aortic valve replacement (TAVI)) via the femoral or transapical approach in those with vascular access problems. Preimplantation balloon aortic valvuloplasty is required and the procedure is usually carried out under general anaesthesia.
- Outcome data for TAVI are difficult to interpret, but in experienced units a 30-day mortality of 8–10% with a stroke rate of 3–4% has been reported. For those patients who survive, haemodynamic and symptomatic improvement appears excellent and there has been no late failure of any device thus far (the longest follow-up of TAVI is now approaching five years).
- At present TAVI it is reserved for patients who are considered too high risk for conventional open AVR. The current indications include a euroSCORE of >20 (euroScore scoring system; www.euroscore.org) or the patient being turned down for surgery (ideally by two surgeons). The National Institute for Health and Clinical Excellence guidelines (NICE 2008) recommend that patient selection should be carried out by a multidisciplinary team including an interventional cardiologist, a cardiac surgeon, and a cardiac anaesthetist. We also encourage involvement of a specialist in care of the elderly and a comprehensive geriatric assessment (see Chapter 12).
- TAVI is not a replacement for aortic valve surgery, which has excellent results. However, many patients are excluded from surgery because of co-morbidities and TAVI is a useful option in this group.

Aortic regurgitation

- Aortic regurgitation (AR) occurs relatively rarely in isolation in the very elderly (>80).
- Usually it is the result of long-standing hypertension or degeneration of an aortic bioprosthesis.
- Less common causes include bacterial endocarditis, aortic dissection, syphilis, Marfan's syndrome, and collagen vascular disease.
- A small number of patients may have combined stenosis and regurgitation and management is then directed to the most severe lesion.

Symptoms and signs
See Table 3.1.

Investigations

ECG: May show LVH.

CXR: May show dilatation of the aortic root and in severe disease cardiomegaly and signs of heart failure.

Doppler echocardiography: Can help estimate the severity as well as provide information on left ventricular dimensions, aortic root dimensions, and left ventricular function.

Management of AR
(See Fig. 3.4.)
- Patients with AR who are candidates for surgical intervention should have echocardiography at regular intervals (at least annually) to detect changes in chamber size.
- Medical treatment with vasodilators such as ACE inhibitors and good blood pressure control is often successful at delaying progression.
- In younger patients (<80 years) prophylactic surgery is advised for those with signs of early left ventricular dysfunction, increasing left ventricular dimensions (end-systolic dimension of >5.5 cm) or diameter of the ascending aorta exceeding 6 cm. In patients over 80 years it is usually deferred to when symptoms occur and patients are otherwise suitable candidates for surgery (see Valve surgery in the elderly, p. 64).
- Emergency surgery for endocarditis or dissection is associated with very high mortality in the elderly, and close liaison between physicians and surgeons is essential to determine the most appropriate intervention.

Mitral regurgitation

- Chronic mitral regurgitation (MR) is the second most common valve disorder in elderly patients.
- It is usually due to myxomatous degeneration of the valve, ischaemic dysfunction of the left ventricle or valvular apparatus, or secondary to dilatation of the left ventricle.
- Less common causes of MR include bacterial endocarditis and collagen vascular disease.
- Acute MR as a result of acute myocardial ischaemia or endocarditis is poorly tolerated and may require emergency surgery if the patient is fit enough. Close liaison between physicians and surgeons is essential here.

Symptoms and signs of MR

Patients may remain asymptomatic for long periods. When symptoms occur they are typical of left ventricular failure: dyspnoea on exertion, orthopnoea, and paroxysmal nocturnal dyspnoea. The characteristic murmur is a loud apical pansystolic murmur. The presence of a third heart sound usually indicates that the lesion is severe. Signs of left ventricular dilatation and left ventricular failure may be present in decompensated patients.

Investigations

ECG: May show evidence of associated ischaemic heart disease.

CXR: May be normal but may show cardiomegaly, left atrial enlargement, and signs of heart failure.

Doppler echocardiography: Provides assessment of the degree of regurgitation, the underlying pathology (dilatation of the valve annulus, ischaemic left ventricular dysfunction, mitral valve prolapse, etc.) as well as information on left ventricular dimensions and function. Serial studies allow assessment of progression.

Management of MR

(See Fig. 3.5.)
- Medical treatment with vasodilators such as ACE inhibitors may be successful at delaying the progression.
- Surgery for MR is indicated in elderly patients with significant symptoms in spite of medical therapy, provided they are suitable for surgery (see Valve surgery in the elderly, p. 64).
- Elderly patients with heart failure should be managed as outlined in Chapter 5.

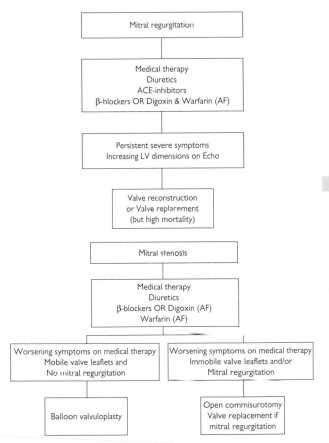

Fig. 3.5 Management of mitral valve disease. ACE, angiotensin-converting enzyme; AF, atrial fibrillation.

Important points to note in surgery for MR in elderly patients

- Repair is generally preferred and provides superior results than replacement.
- Mild residual regurgitation after repair is acceptable.
- Severe annular calcification is an additional risk for valve replacement.
- Bioprostheses are more difficult to implant in the mitral position and their superiority over mechanical prostheses is marginal.
- Functional regurgitation in ischaemic cardiomyopathy often improves with myocardial revascularization without the need for additional valve surgery.

Outcome of mitral valve surgery in the elderly

Mitral valve replacement is less well tolerated than AVR. The mortality rate in octogenarians is between 10% and 20%, and survival rates are 80%, 64%, and 41% at one, three, and five years, respectively. The impact of valve repair on survival and quality of life in octogenarians is currently unknown because of the small number of patients reported.

A transvenous catheter-delivered implantable device to provide a percutaneous alternative to surgical mitral annuloplasty has been developed. Initial experience shows it is feasible and results are favourable. This technique requires further evaluation as a less invasive alternative to surgical annuloplasty.

Mitral stenosis

Mitral stenosis (MS) is an uncommon condition in the elderly, and mainly caused by rheumatic heart disease. Mitral annulus calcification rarely causes significant MS.

Symptoms and signs in MS

Patients with MS may be asymptomatic for many years. Symptoms result from increased left atrial pressure and reduced cardiac output, and although left ventricular contractility is normal, symptoms are usually typical of left-sided heart failure: dyspnoea on exertion, orthopnoea, and paroxysmal nocturnal dyspnoea. Haemoptysis, hoarseness, and symptoms of right heart failure are less frequent but more specific. Systemic embolisation may be the first manifestation.

The clinical diagnosis may be difficult to establish, due to the absence of the usual physical signs, especially if cardiac output is low (silent MS). Characteristic findings are a loud first heart sound and a low-pitched diastolic rumble that follows an opening snap. Signs of pulmonary hypertension (loud P2 and parasternal lift) and right ventricular overload indicate pulmonary hypertension, which increases the risk of surgery.

Investigations

ECG – may show p mitrale in sinus rhythm.

CXR – shows left atrial enlargement and in severe disease may show cardiomegaly due to right ventricular enlargement and signs of pulmonary oedema.

Doppler echocardiography – allows accurate assessment of the severity of stenosis as well as detecting the presence of significant calcification and associated mitral regurgitation. The latter two factors are important in determining treatment options.

Treatment

- Diuretics are usually effective at reducing left atrial pressure and reducing dyspnoea.
- Because of the high risk of systemic embolization, especially in those with atrial fibrillation or a dilated left atrium, anticoagulation with warfarin is indicated in most patients with MS.
- When atrial fibrillation occurs, rate control is important as a rapid heart rate will further impair left ventricular filling and increase symptoms. Most patients will require a β-blocker or rate-slowing calcium channel blocker ± digoxin (see Chapter 7) to achieve adequate rate control.
- Surgery is indicated for symptomatic patients and often requires replacement of the valve, as repair is often not possible due to rigid and calcified valvular components. Symptoms are seldom severe until the valve area is 1 cm^2 or less.
- A mechanical prosthesis is generally recommended, as most of these patients require anticoagulation to reduce the risk of systemic embolization.

- Percutaneous balloon commissurotomy is an alternative to surgery in high-risk patients with predominant stenosis. The procedural mortality in patients over 70 is about 5%, with improved transvalvular haemodynamics in 50%, in the short term. Fifty per cent of patients, however, required surgery within three years so it is not a long-term solution (Prêtre and Turina 2000).

Other conditions causing murmurs in the elderly

Hypertrophic cardiomyopathy

Hypertrophic cardiomyopathy is often thought to be predominantly a disease of younger patients. However, wide phenotypic expression of the gene abnormality is recognized and some patients may survive relatively free of symptoms into old age. Symptoms of outflow tract obstruction may develop in the elderly and are similar to those of aortic valve stenosis, namely, syncope, dizziness, palpitation, dyspnoea, and chest pain. The murmur may be difficult to distinguish from that of AS and/or MR. Doppler echocardiography provides confirmation of the diagnosis. Referral to a cardiologist is recommended for advice on treatment options, investigations, and familial screening.

Atrial septal defect

A congenital atrial septal defect (ASD) can occasionally present for the first time in the elderly. Significant ASDs are associated with increased morbidity and mortality. Elderly ASD patients frequently have reduced exercise capacity, arrhythmias (most commonly atrial fibrillation), pulmonary hypertension, and concomitant cardiac and extracardiac pathology, including ischemic heart disease, diabetes, and lung disease.

The results of trials of surgical ASD closure with regard to mortality and morbidity are controversial, with some showing increased mortality. Recent studies show that percutaneous closure is possible in elderly patients but the long-term effects on mortality and morbidity are unclear. Referral to a specialist centre with experience in the elderly is recommended in symptomatic patients.

Tricuspid regurgitation

Tricuspid regurgitation (TR) in the elderly is most often caused by dilatation of the valve ring secondary to right ventricular failure, usually resulting from left-sided heart failure or pulmonary hypertension related to primary lung disease. Infective endocarditis is a rare cause.

TR may be silent, or a short ejection or pansystolic murmur may be heard in the third or fourth intercostal space at the left sternal border. The murmur increases in intensity with inspiration (Carvallo's sign). If TR is severe, a prominent v wave may be seen in the jugular venous pulse. The diagnosis is confirmed by Doppler echocardiography.

Medical treatment of heart failure ameliorates TR. Surgery is rarely necessary.

Valve surgery in the elderly

- The ability of elderly patients to withstand cardiac surgery is reduced due to co-morbidities (Table 3.2), reduced functional reserve of vital organs, and diminished defence and adaptation capacities.
- There are substantial discrepancies on an individual level between chronological and physiological age.
- With improvements in operative techniques, perioperative, and postoperative care, mortality and morbidity from heart surgery has declined in all age groups, and more elderly patients are now considered candidates for cardiac surgery.
- Atheroma of aorta is frequent in elderly patients and increases risk of embolization and neurological deficits post operatively.
- Cerebral hypoperfusion as a result of atherosclerosis and impaired cerebral autoregulation may result in global or local hypoperfusion of the brain. This can lead to delayed awakening, agitation, and incomplete return of cognitive function. Diffuse and focal neurological deficits may affect 15–20% of elderly patients after heart surgery, leading to prolonged hospital stay, increasing dependence, or death.

Table 3.2 Common co-morbidities in octogenarians with valve disease

Coronary artery disease	40–60%
Obstructive lung disease	15–25%
Renal insufficiency	5–10%
Peripheral vascular disease	2–10%
Cerebrovascular disease	5–25%
Hypertension	20–50%
Diabetes	10–20%

Factors to consider in assessing risk

There are a number of different risk stratification models (e.g. EuroSCORE (www.euroscore.org) and Parsonnet (www.mpoullis.com/Parsonnet.htm)) for assessing operative mortality in cardiac surgery, but they all have limitations. Important factors to consider in the elderly are:

- *Age:* Appears in all scoring systems as an incremental risk factor for postoperative mortality, however, the true influence of age is difficult to estimate, because of the high prevalence of other confounding factors. Age alone should not be a determining factor. In those over 80, surgery should be considered only in symptomatic patients where it is likely to improve their quality of life.

- **Type of operation:** AVR for AS is a well established and tolerated operation in the elderly including octogenarians, and therefore should be considered particular in symptomatic patients. The additional need for CABG or mitral valve repair or replacement increases the operative risk. In some elderly patients, a technically and physiologically less demanding operation may be performed, after discussion with the patient, at the cost of an incomplete repair, with reduced long-term benefit but improved symptom control.
- **Presence of significant co-morbidities:** Co-morbidities that are frequent in the elderly and likely to affect the outcome of surgery are listed in Table 3.2. In general the more severe the condition the greater is its effect. Relative contraindications to surgery especially in those over 80 years are listed in Table 3.3.
- **Patients' views:** Patient preference is important to consider and some patients may decline surgery even though they realise this may shorten their lifespan. The physical and emotional trauma involved in cardiac surgery can be considerable and may deter an elderly patient from accepting surgery. It is very important to involve the patient in all discussions and respect their views.

Table 3.3 Contraindications to valve surgery in the elderly

Coronary artery disease and left ventricular ejection fraction <30%
Creatinine >200 μmol/l
Chronic obstructive pulmonary disease with forced expiratory volume in one second (FEV$_1$) <800 ml
Neurological or physical disease restricting the patient's independence, outside activity, or both
Significant psychiatric disorders (dementia, severe depression)
Cancer or other condition reducing quality of life, survival, or both

Preoperative assessment

Prior to considering valve surgery, all patients should have:
- Assessment of cardiorespiratory function (echocardiogram and pulmonary function tests)
- Assessment of renal function
- Neurological and physical assessment including the metabolic equivalent of activities of daily living (METs) (see Chapter 12)
- Cognitive assessment (Mini-Mental State Examination)
- Coronary angiography: 40–60% of patients with valve disease have associated coronary artery disease, which will influence the outcome of surgery. Appropriate revascularization is beneficial in the elderly. The risk of angiography does increase with age (mortality of 0.5% in >80 years) but the information obtained is helpful in determining not only the risk of but also the most appropriate operation to be performed.

- Carotid Doppler ultrasound is recommended to reduce the risk of postoperative stroke. For symptomatic or bilateral high-grade stenosis, carotid endarterectomy before or at the time of heart surgery should be considered. In those with an asymptomatic stenosis or occlusion, care should be taken to ensure higher perfusion pressures perioperatively.
- We recommend a Comprehensive Geriatric Assessment (CGA) as employed by the **Proactive Care of Older People undergoing surgery (POPS) project** (see Chapter 12). This should address many of these issues and also help plan discharge and recovery after surgery by early involvement of appropriate services.

Important points to remember

- Valvular heart disease is responsible for a significant proportion of mortality and morbidity in the elderly.
- Calcific aortic stenosis is the most common valve lesion seen, and the results from valve surgery are good even in octogenarians.
- The presentation and manifestation of valvular heart disease often differ from those in younger patients. The initial clinical picture may be non-specific, and other pathological processes and age-related changes often obscure the diagnosis.
- Non-invasive Doppler echocardiographic techniques allow accurate assessment of valve lesions.
- Management of valve disease in the elderly is complex and the decision for surgery a difficult one involving medical, ethical, and social issues.

Guidelines, references, and recommended reading

American College of Cardiology/American Hearth Association (2008) ACC/AHA practice guideline: 2008 focused update incorporated into the ACC/AHA 2006 Guidelines for the Management of Patients with Valvular Heart Disease. *J Am Coll Cardiol* **52**:1–142. Available at: www.americanheart.org.

Anon (2007) Guidelines on the management of valvular heart disease. The Task Force on the Management of Valvular Heart Disease of the European Society of Cardiology. *Eur Heart J* **28**: 230–68. Available at: www.escardio.org/guidelines.

Ellis G and Langhorne P. Comprehensive geriatric assessment for older hospital patients. Br Med Bull, 2005, **71**:45–49.

euroScore scoring system. Available at: www.euroscore.org

Harari D, Hopper A, Dhesi J, Babic-Illman G, Lockwood L, Finbarr M. (2007) Proactive Care of older people undergoing surgery (POPS): Designing, embedding, evaluating and funding a comprehensive assessment service for older elective surgical patients. *Age Ageing* **36**:190–6.

National Institute for Health and Clinical Excellence. (2008) Transcatheter aortic valve implantation for aortic stenosis. IPG 266. London: National Institute for Health and Clinical Excellence. Available at: www.nice.org.uk/ipg266

Prêtre R, Turina MI (2000) Valve disease: cardiac valve surgery in the octogenarian. *Heart* **83**:116–21.

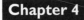
Infective endocarditis

Introduction

- Infection of the endothelial lining of the heart.
- High incidence in elderly population compared with the general population.
- More common in males than females.
- Mortality ~25% and higher in the elderly than in younger patients.
- Evolving disease pattern due to change in infective organisms, antibiotic therapy and pre-existing cardiac disease.
- Increasing use of the device therapy (pacemakers and intracardiac defibrillators) in elderly patients has led to increased risk of infection of these devices.

Pathogenesis

Figure 4.1 gives a schematic overview of the pathogenesis of infective endocarditis.

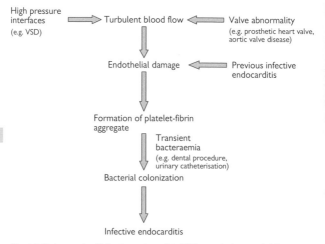

Fig. 4.1 Pathogenesis of infective endocarditis. VSD, ventricular septal defect.

Risk factors for infective endocarditis (Fig. 4.2)

Cardiac disease	Immunosuppression	Other
Prosthetic heart valve	Chronic disease	Diabetes mellitus
Previous infective endocarditis	Steroid therapy	Gastrointestinal cancer
Aortic valve disease	Haemodialysis	Genitourinary cancer
Mitral regurgitation	Human immunode-ficiency virus (HIV) infection	Dental work/poor dental hygiene
Degenerative valve disease		Recent central line
Ischaemic heart disease		Intravenous drug use
Ventricular septal defect		
Rheumatic heart disease		
Mural thrombus		
Permanent pacemaker or implantable cardiac defibrillator		

Fig. 4.2 Risk factors for infective endocarditis.
■ Major predisposing conditions in elderly population when compared with the younger population (Durante-Mangoni et al. 2008).
■ More common in elderly population when compared with the younger population.

Presentation

The presentation of infective endocarditis is often non-specific in the elderly; it is therefore important to have a high index of suspicion. Symptoms and signs arise from the infection itself, cardiac manifestations or complications (e.g. immune complex disease, embolic disease).

Symptoms

- Malaise
- Lethargy
- Fever
- Weight loss
- Anorexia
- Night sweats
- Headaches
- Arthralgia
- Myalgia
- Confusion
- Falls
- Palpitations
- Chest pain
- Collapse
- Shortness of breath
- Focal neurological deficit
- Left upper quadrant pain.

Signs

- Fever (not always present in elderly patients with infective endocarditis)
- Pallor
- Confusion
- Murmur – new or changing
- Tachycardia
- Evidence of congestive cardiac failure (CCF)
- Petechiae – conjunctival, buccal, palatal, skin
- Clubbing
- Splinter haemorrhages
- Osler's nodes on finger pulps
- Janeway lesions on palms and/or soles
- Roth spots or retinal haemorrhage on fundoscopy
- Splenomegaly
- Focal neurological deficit
- Infarction of extremities
- Abdominal tenderness due to kidney, bowel or splenic infarction.

Investigations

Investigation	Result associated with infective endocarditis
Urine dipstick	Haematuria, proteinuria
Full blood count	Mild/moderate normocytic anaemia, ↑/normal WCC, ↓/normal platelet count
C-reactive protein (CRP)	↑
Erythrocyte sedimentation rate (ESR)	↑
Serum protein electrophoresis	↑ gamma-globulins
Rheumatoid factor	Positive (may return to negative once treated)
Complement (C3, C4)	↓/normal
≥ 3 × Blood cultures	Positive
Electrocardiogram (ECG)	Conduction defects, e.g. heart block
Chest radiograph (CXR)	May suggest heart failure
Echocardiogram	Transthoracic (TTE) initially, transoesophageal if TTE negative or suspected myocardial abscess/ perivalvular extension

Duke criteria

- Collection of criteria that can be used to establish a diagnosis of infective endocarditis.
- 80–90% sensitive
- Diagnosis can be made if any of the following three combinations of criteria are present (Table 4.1):
  - Two major
  - One major + three minor
  - Five minor.

Table 4.1 Duke criteria for establishing diagnosis of infective endocarditis

Major criteria	Minor criteria
Positive blood culture ×2 with a typical infective endocarditis organism (see Organisms causing infective endocarditis in elderly patients, p. 78)	Fever >38°C
Endocardial involvement demonstrated on echo, e.g. vegetation, abscess, prosthetic valve dehiscence, new valvular regurgitation	Predisposing factor – known cardiac lesion
	Evidence of embolism, e.g. Janeway lesions, conjunctival haemorrhage
	Immune complex disease, e.g. glomerulonephritis, positive rheumatoid factor
	Positive blood culture (that does not meet major criteria)
	Positive echo (that does not meet major criteria)
	Serology consistent with infective endocarditis

Organisms causing infective endocarditis in elderly patients

- *Staphylococcus aureus* – incidence increasing
- *Streptococcus viridans* – less common in elderly population compared with the general population
- *Streptococcus bovis* – more common in elderly population compared with general population; related to higher incidence of gastrointestinal pathology
- Enterococci – related to higher incidence of gastrointestinal and genitourinary pathology in elderly population
- Organisms from the HACEK group (*Haemophilus* species (excluding *Haemophilus influenzae*), *Actinobacillus actinomycetemcomitans, Cardiobacterium hominis, Eikenella corrodens, Kingella kingae*)
- *Coxiella**
- *Legionella**
- *Yeasts**

*Atypical according to Duke criteria.

Elderly patients have a higher blood culture yield than younger patients. However, if the patient has had antibiotic treatment before blood cultures are taken, they may not be positive. Other causes of negative blood cultures include infection with fastidious organisms (require longer incubation) or infection with yeasts. Polymerase chain reaction and serology can be used to identify organisms that are not readily cultured.

Complications

Local

- Heart failure
- Conduction abnormalities – most common if infection involves aortic ring
- Mycotic aneurysm of proximal aorta or coronary arteries.

Other

- Embolization of vegetations → limb ischaemia, pneumonia, splenic infarcts, bowel ischaemia
- Stroke – due to infarction (embolism) or haemorrhage (cerebral mycotic aneurysm)
- Immune complex disease → vasculitic rash, arthritis, glomerulonephritis
- Complications of treatment, e.g. antibiotic sensitivity, renal impairment.

Treatment

- Choice of antibiotic therapy depends on organisms isolated from blood cultures.
- Involve microbiology team from an early stage; consult local guidelines.
- Antibiotics should be administered intravenously – affected areas often do not have blood supply, but come into contact with blood as it passes through heart, allowing the antibiotics to diffuse into vegetations.
- If the patient is unwell due to sepsis, do not withhold antibiotic therapy until culture results are available.
- Common regimen for sensitive organisms is combination of penicillin and aminoglycoside (e.g. gentamicin), which are bactericidal.
- Usually require 4–6 weeks of treatment to ensure eradication of infecting organism. Duration of treatment depends on infecting organism and presence of prosthetic valves, etc and needs to be determined for each patient depending on the response to treatment.
- Indications for surgery are similar to those in younger patients and include severe heart failure not responding to medical treatment, prosthetic dehiscence, valvular obstruction, periannular or myocardial abscess or multiple emboli, and persistent infection in spite of antibiotic therapy. Close collaboration between surgeons, physicians and microbiologists is essential in caring for there patients. Evidence shows that elderly patients are less likely to be referred for surgery but the outcome in those who have surgery is similar to that in younger patients so they should be considered for surgery.
- In patient with infected devices the device should be removed as soon as is feasible and antibiotics administered according to sensitivities. A new device should not be inserted until infection has resolved.
- Treatment also involves monitoring for and managing delirium, pressure sore prevention and management, and ensuring adequate hydration and nutrition. Early referral to the dietician is recommended.
- In patients with who are likely to require intravenous therapy for greater than two weeks, early referral for a peripherally inserted central line (PICC) (for antibiotic administration and blood tests) will facilitate management.
- Elderly patients with infective endocarditis comprise a high-risk group and usually require inpatient treatment for several weeks. (See the European Society of Cardiology guidelines for recommendations for home antibiotic therapy (Task Force 2009).) Considerable psychological and physical stress can result, and it is important to address this. Involve the multidisciplinary team early to help keep the patient motivated and as mobile as possible. This will facilitate return to the community at the end of treatment. A period of rehabilitation either as an inpatient or in the community, depending on local availability, may be required, and early discharge planning is essential.

Prophylaxis

The National Institute for Health and Clinical Excellence (NICE) guidelines for prophylaxis against infective endocarditis were published in 2008. The most notable recommendation is that patients at risk of developing infective endocarditis should no longer be given antibiotic prophylaxis when having interventional procedures. This guidance was based on a lack of efficacy of antibiotic prophylaxis regimens, a lack of association between infective endocarditis episodes and prior interventional procedures, a recognition of the prevalence of everyday activities (such as toothbrushing) resulting in bacteraemias, and an appreciation of the risks involved in antibiotic prophylaxis (e.g. anaphylaxis).

Summary of the NICE guidelines

- Patients at risk should be advised to maintain good oral health.
- Patients at risk should be given information regarding the risks of undergoing invasive procedures and the symptoms of infective endocarditis.
- Antibiotic prophylaxis is **not** recommended for dental procedures, gastrointestinal tract procedures, genitourinary tract procedures, bronchoscopy, or respiratory tract infections.
- Patients at risk of infective endocarditis who have infection should be investigated promptly and treated with appropriate antibiotics.

There is still some controversy regarding the NICE guidelines. Some cardiologists still recommend prophylaxis in high-risk groups (e.g. prosthetic valves and those with previous episode of endocarditis) so it is best to check if there is a local policy. Other recent guidelines are available from the American Heart Association (2007) and the British Society of Antimicrobial Chemotherapy (BSAC) (2006). Advice on the antibiotics to use should be obtained from local microbiologists or the BSAC guidelines.

Guidelines, references, and recommended reading

Durante-Mangoni E, Bradley S, Selton-Suty C, Tripodi MF, Barsic B, Bouza E, et al.; International Collaboration on Endocarditis Prospective Cohort Study Group (2008) Current features of infective endocarditis in elderly patients. Arch Intern Med **168**:2095–2103.

Gould FK, Elliot TS, Foweraker J, Fulford M, Perry JD, Roberts GJ, et al. (2006) Guidelines for the prevention of endocarditis: report of the Working Party of the British Society for Antimicrobial Chemotherapy. J Antimicrob Chemother **57**:1035–42.

National Institute for Health and Clinical Excellence (2007) Prophylaxis against infective endocarditis: antimicrobial prophylaxis against infective endocarditis in adults and children undergoing interventional procedures. Clinical guideline 64. London: National Institute for Health and Clinical Excellence. Available at: www.nice.org.uk/cg64.

Prendergast B (2006) The changing face of infective endocarditis. Heart **92**:879–85.

Guidelines on the prevention, diagnosis, and treatment of infective endocarditis (new version 2009): the Task Force on the Prevention, Diagnosis, and Treatment of Infective Endocarditis of the European Society of Cardiology (ESC). Eur Heart J **30**:2369–413. Available at: www. escardio.org/guidelines.

Wilson W, Taubert KA, Gewitz M, Lockhart PB, Baddour LM, Levison M, et al. (2007) Prevention of infective endocarditis. Guidelines from the American Heart Association. Circulation **116**: 1736–54. Available at: www.americanheart.org.

Heart failure

Chronic heart failure

Epidemiology

- Incidence and prevalence increase with increasing age; average age at diagnosis is 76.
- 1/15 of those >75 years; doubles in those >85 years; increasingly common as population ages and survival from myocardial infarction (MI) improves.
- Risk of heart failure is higher in men at all ages, but more women have heart failure due to population demographics.
- Accounts for 5% of all emergency medical admissions to hospital and 2% of all National Health Service (NHS) inpatient bed days. This is predicted to rise by 50% in next 25 years due to ageing of the population.
- High rate of mortality; 50% die within 4 years of diagnosis.
- 40% with heart failure admitted to hospital are dead or readmitted within 1 year.

Definition

Heart failure is a complex syndrome and difficult to define. It results from any structural or functional cardiac disorder that impairs the ability of the heart to function as a pump to support a physiological circulation. The European Society of Cardiology (ESC) gives a more clinical definition which includes diagnostic features.

Heart failure is a clinical syndrome in which patients have the following features:

- Symptoms typical of heart failure (breathlessness at rest or on exercise, fatigue, tiredness, ankle swelling)

and

- Signs typical of heart failure (tachycardia, tachypnoea, pulmonary crackles, pleural effusion, raised jugular venous pressure (JVP), peripheral oedema, hepatomegaly)

and

- Objective evidence of a structural or functional abnormality at rest (cardiomegaly, third heart sound, murmur, abnormality on Echo, raised natriuretic peptide concentration).

Source: ESC guidelines (2008).

Commonest cause in the UK is coronary heart disease (contributing to 70%), followed by hypertension and tachyarrhythmias (often atrial fibrillation (AF)). Other cardiorespiratory causes include:
- Valvular disease
- Pericardial disease
- Pulmonary hypertension.

Most other causes reflect disease of the heart muscle. Those most relevant in the elderly include:

- Cardiomyopathies
- Toxins: alcohol, anthracycline chemotherapy
- Nutritional: deficiency of thiamine (beriberi), selenium, obesity, and cachexia
- Infiltrative: sarcoidosis, amyloidosis, connective tissue disease.

In addition, diseases which result in an increase in cardiac output beyond the left ventricle's capability can cause it to fail. Examples of 'high output' states are: anaemia, thyrotoxicosis, and Paget's disease. Heart failure should resolve with treatment of the underlying diagnosis.

Symptoms and signs

Symptoms

Breathlessness, fatigue, and fluid retention are characteristic symptoms, but presentation may be more vague in elderly patients. Fatigue alone may be the predominant symptom. In severe cases cachexia may result.

Breathlessness is used as the basis of the New York Heart Association (NYHA) classification of severity in heart failure (Table 5.1). The classification can be used to monitor effectiveness of treatment and is often referenced in clinical trials.

Table 5.1 New York Heart Association (NYHA) classification of severity of breathlessness in heart failure

NYHA class	Patient symptoms
Class I (mild)	No limitation of physical activity. Ordinary physical activity does not cause undue fatigue, palpitation, or dyspnoea
Class II (mild)	Slight limitation of physical activity. Comfortable at rest but ordinary physical activity results in undue fatigue, palpitation, or dyspnoea
Class III (moderate)	Marked limitation of physical activity. Less than ordinary physical activity results in undue fatigue, palpitation, or dyspnoea
Class IV (severe)	Dyspnoea present at rest. Unable to carry out any physical activity without discomfort

No one symptom is diagnostic of heart failure and alternative diagnoses should always be considered if the clinical picture is unclear.

Signs

When assessing the elderly patient a combination of some of the signs shown in Table 5.2, in conjunction with suggestive symptoms, should lead to further investigation for heart failure.

Table 5.2 Signs of heart failure

Examination	Findings
Pulse	Tachycardic
	Often low volume
	May be irregular
Fluid status	Increased weight
	Raised JVP
	Peripheral oedema (see Box 5.1 for differential diagnosis in the elderly)
	Sacral oedema
Respiratory	Raised respiratory rate
	Crackles
	Pleural effusions
Cardiovascular	Displaced apex
	Third heart sound
	Gallop rhythm
	Murmurs suggesting valvular dysfunction
Abdominal	Hepatomegaly
	Ascites

Box 5.1 The differential diagnosis of ankle oedema in the elderly: it may not be heart failure

- Medications: non-steroidal anti-inflammatory drugs (NSAIDs), amlodipine.
- Peripheral venous insufficiency: usually accompanied by overlying chronic skin changes such as venous eczema. Leg elevation when sitting and sleeping may help (although a diuresis may result).
- Secondary to acute thrombophlebitis or cellulitis: the leg will be painful and erythematous.
- Low serum albumin: gastrointestinal loss, sepsis, chronic disease, nephrotic syndrome.
- Obstruction of lymphatic drainage: examine the abdomen for pelvic tumours and the inguinal regions for lymphadenopathy.
- Always consider DVT if swelling appears more unilateral.

Diagnosis and investigation

'Heart failure' is not a diagnosis. Clinical diagnosis alone is especially inaccurate in women, the obese, and the elderly. The key diagnostic tests are non-invasive and should be tolerated well by elderly patients. Clinical assessment and investigations should aim to establish a cause and characterize the extent of ventricular impairment.

Electrocardiogram (ECG)

Look for:
- Signs of previous ischaemia: Q waves, poor R wave progression, ST/T segment changes
- Signs of conduction abnormalities: bundle branch block (Fig. 5.1), AF
- Signs of hypertension: left ventricular hypertrophy (LVH).

Chest radiograph (CXR)

Look for:
- Cardiomegaly (Fig. 5.2)
- Extra fluid: upper lobe blood diversion, 'bat wing' pulmonary oedema, Kerley B lines, pleural effusions
- Alternative causes of breathlessness.

(Heart failure is extremely unlikely if ECG and CXR are normal).

Blood tests

- Look for reversible causes: anaemia, thyroid function.
- Consider secondary prevention: glucose, lipids.
- Establish baseline renal function and electrolytes before commencing therapy.
- Liver function tests may be deranged in hepatic congestion.
- Measure B-type natriuretic peptide (BNP) (see Box 5.2).

Box 5.2 Natriuretic peptides

- BNP and N-terminal pro-BNP (NT-proBNP) are used as diagnostic and management tools in heart failure.
- They rise in response to increased myocardial wall stress.
- A normal concentration in an untreated patient has a high negative predictive value and makes heart failure an unlikely diagnosis.
- A raised concentration does not confirm heart failure; LVH, tachycardia, hypoxaemia, renal dysfunction, sepsis, and advanced age can all cause levels to rise.
- Natriuretic peptides can also be used to monitor response to treatment; high levels despite optimal therapy in heart failure indicate a poor prognosis.

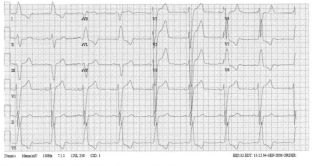

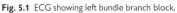

Fig. 5.1 ECG showing left bundle branch block.

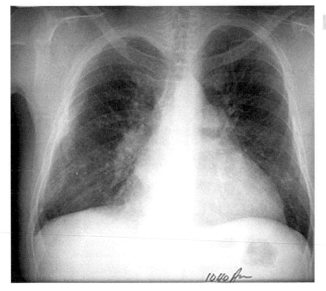

Fig. 5.2 CXR showing cardiomegaly and pulmonary oedema.

Echo

Transthoracic Doppler two-dimensional (2D) echocardiography is used to assess systolic function of the left ventricle. It is possible to determine the cause of heart failure in many cases: regional wall motion abnormalities suggest ischaemia, valve disease, LVH secondary to hypertension, dilated cardiomyopathy, e.g. secondary to alcohol, pericardial disease (rare) and evidence of infiltration secondary to, e.g., amyloid.

Rarely further investigation may be needed if the above investigations are inconclusive but the diagnosis is still clinically likely:

- Cardiac magnetic resonance imaging: sometimes not tolerated by patients in this age group. May be contraindicated if patient has an implanted device or other implant such as joint replacement.
- Radionuclide imaging: may be useful in determining cause and myocardial viability.
- Cardiac catheterization: diagnostic and therapeutic potential but much more invasive.

Other tests may also be needed to explore alternative diagnoses, e.g. pulmonary function tests. In the UK, the National Institute for Health and Clinical Excellence (NICE 2003) has suggested the diagnostic algorithm shown in Figure 5.3.

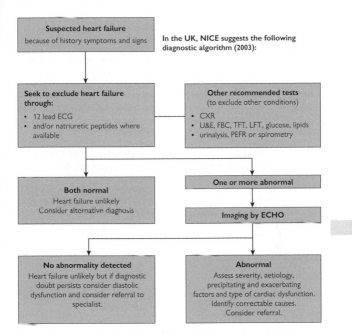

Fig. 5.3 Diagnostic algorithm for heart failure. CXR, chest radiograph; U+Es, urea and electrolytes; FBC, full blood count; TFT, thyroid function test; LFT, liver function test; PEFR, peak expiratory flow rate. (Adapted from: National Collaborating Centre for Chronic Conditions. *Chronic heart failure: national clinical guideline for diagnosis and management in primary and secondary care.* London, RCP: 2003. Copyright © 2003 Royal College of Physicians. Reproduced by permission).

Heart failure with preserved systolic function

Definition

A clinical syndrome of cardiac failure with preserved left ventricular ejection fraction (LVEF) on echo and no significant valvular disease.

Also known as: diastolic heart failure, heart failure with preserved ejection fraction (HFPEF), heart failure with normal ejection fraction (HFNEF).

Epidemiology

- 50% of patients with clinical evidence of heart failure have HFPEF.
- More common in elderly (mean age 74–76 years) and females (>60%).
- High all-cause mortality after hospitalization for heart failure. Current evidence is that non-heart failure cardiovascular mortality is higher in this group than in patients with heart failure and systolic dysfunction:
  - 2.9% in-hospital mortality
  - 22–29% 1-year mortality
  - 65% 5-year morality.
- Associated co-morbidities are frequent and likely to affect morbidity and mortality:
  - Hypertension (>70%)
  - Coronary artery disease (CHD) (30–50%)
  - AF (30–40%)
  - Diabetes mellitus (35–50%)
  - Chronic kidney disease (25%)
  - Cerebrovascular disease (15%).

Diagnosis

Diagnosis requires that three criteria are satisfied:

- Presence of signs and/or symptoms of chronic heart failure.
- Presence of normal left ventricular systolic function (LVEF >50%).
- Evidence of diastolic dysfunction: abnormal left ventricular relaxation or diastolic stiffness.

Management

- No treatment has yet been shown to convincingly reduce morbidity and mortality in this patient group.
- The mainstay of therapy is presently good control of blood pressure in all patients and of ventricular rate in those with AF.
- Diuretics may also be used for symptomatic relief.

Two large trials have suggested that angiotensin receptor blockers (ARBs) (candesartan in the CHARM preserved trial) and angiotensin-converting enzyme (ACE) inhibitors (perindopril in the PEP-CHF trial) may reduce hospitalization in patients with HFPEV. Other trials of ARBs are less promising (see Chapter 11). We would recommend their use especially if symptoms persist in spite of diuretics and to control blood pressure in hypertension.

As for all patients with cardiovascular disease, secondary prevention is extremely important. Dietary and lifestyle advice should be offered and help given to stop smoking. Patients should be prescribed 75 mg aspirin unless contraindicated and appropriate lipid-lowering therapy.

Treatment of systolic heart failure

Ideally the treatment of heart failure should be delivered by a multidisciplinary team encompassing a general practitioner, heart failure nurse, cardiologist, and ultimately community palliative care services. Treatment should consist of a non-pharmacological as well as pharmacological approach. Any reversible causes discovered during initial investigation should also be corrected.

Non-pharmacological treatments

Patient education

This can pose particular problems in those with cognitive impairment, but every effort should be made to explain the diagnosis, prognosis, and medication. The opportunity should be taken to ensure the patient has realistic expectations regarding response to treatment and possible side effects of tablets. Time spent with patients and their carers early in diagnosis will increase concordance with medications and facilitate more difficult end-of-life decisions when they arise.

Lifestyle changes

Patients should be advised about the following lifestyle changes. If the patient does not prepare their own meals, speak to their care provider or the manager of their care facility:

• Decrease sodium intake: no quantitative guideline exists but excessive salt intake should be avoided. A dietician can advise on the salt content of common foods.
• Those with severe heart failure or hyponatraemia may benefit from fluid restriction of 1.5 l/day.
• Limit alcohol intake to 1–2 units/day. Any patient with alcohol-induced cardiomyopathy should abstain completely.
• Stop smoking: may need referral to specialist services.
• Supervised exercise training programmes have proven benefit and should be encouraged in the elderly.

Review medication

A number of medications prescribed for other conditions can precipitate or exacerbate heart failure. Some of the common ones are listed in Table 5.3. Regular medication review is essential in heart failure patients at least at 6-monthly intervals (see Table 5.3).

Table 5.3 Drugs to avoid or use with caution in heart failure

Drug class	Effect
Non-steroidal anti-inflammatory drugs (NSAIDs)	Deterioration of symptoms due to systemic vasoconstriction
	Cause renal dysfunction and exacerbate renal dysfunction associated with ACE, ARB and aldosterone antagonists
Corticosteroids	Exacerbate fluid retention
Calcium channel blockers	Except for amlodipine and felodipine they are negatively inotropic and can cause decompensation. Amlodipine and felodipine can worsen peripheral oedema
Cilostazol – a phosphodiesterase inhibitor (used in peripheral vascular disease)	Other phosphodiesterase inhibitors have shown increased mortality in heart failure
Thiazolinediones (e.g. rosiglitazone and pioglitazone)	Cause fluid retention and may worsen heart failure symptoms and signs. Also concern regarding increased cardiovascular risk with rosiglitazone
Phosphodiesterase inhibitors (e.g. sildenafil)	Can cause systemic hypotension and are contraindicated in patients on nitrates
α-Adrenoreceptor antagonists	May exacerbate heart failure and cause symptomatic hypotension and postural hypotension
Aspirin – current guidelines recommend aspirin in patients with coronary artery disease ± heart failure	There is some concern that aspirin may attenuate the beneficial effects of ACE inhibitors so review indication if poor response to ACE inhibitor therapy
Statins – currently recommended in patients with coronary artery disease ± heart failure	Controversial as epidemiological studies show and an association between low cholesterol and poor prognosis. Two recent trials (CORONA and GISSI-HF) show no evidence of mortality benefit but no adverse effect

Cardiac rehabilitation

This has been shown to be beneficial for heart failure patients. Regular physical activity improves exercise tolerance and quality of life, and reduces hospitalization and mortality. Age is not a contraindication so elderly patients should be referred to local rehabilitation programmes unless there are other reasons why they cannot participate, e.g. mobility limited due to osteoarthritis, cognitive impairment, etc. Individualized home-based programmes may be especially suited to the elderly but at present are not widely available. Cost is a factor but the reduction in hospitalization could offset this, so more programmes need to be developed with ease of access for the elderly.

Vaccination
Pneumococcal and influenza vaccination should be a priority in the elderly with heart failure.

Screen for depression
The prevalence of clinically significant depression in heart failure patients may be as high as 20%. Depression is associated with increased morbidity and mortality. The geriatric depression scale can be used as a screening tool and further treatment discussed with the patient if likely depression is detected. See Chapter 14 for guidelines on treatment in patients with cardiovascular disease.

Heart failure nurses
Heart failure nurses provide proven benefit – they can initiate most of the non-pharmacological approaches listed above and can review patients at home and in the community to uptitrate their medications. This can be especially helpful in the elderly, who may find frequent clinic visits for medication titration difficult. They also provide a valuable educational role, which will help improve compliance and concordance.

Pharmacological treatments

The primary outcome measured in most trials of heart failure medication in those with reduced ejection fraction is mortality. However, in reality a reduction in morbidity and improved quality of life is often far more important in the elderly patient group. Drug treatment will be required in most patients with a heart failure diagnosis. The maximum tolerated dose of a drug should be aimed for rather than symptomatic relief alone. Figure 5.4 shows a recommended approach to drug treatment in chronic heart failure and Table 5.4 provides a summary of the drugs used in the treatment of heart failure in elderly patients.

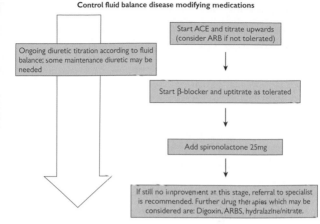

Fig. 5.4 Recommended step-wise approach to drug treatment (see also Table 5.4) for chronic heart failure. In the acute setting fluid balance should be achieved before disease modifying medications are started. ACE, angiotensin-converting enzyme; ARB, angiotensin receptor II antagonist.

If the patient remains symptomatic after optimization of pharmacological therapy implantable devices may be considered (see Device therapy: is there a role in the elderly?, pp.106–8).

Table 5.4 Guide to medications used in treatment of heart failure (dose, side effects and monitoring)

Medication	Suggested dosing in the elderly	Common side effects and suggested action
ACE inhibitors Increase life expectancy Decrease hospitalization E.g.: Ramipril 1.25 mg od; target 5 mg bd Lisinopril 2.5 mg od; target 30–40 mg od	Start at lowest dose and double the dose at not less than fortnightly intervals Check U+Es at baseline and after 1–2 weeks. Recheck 1–2 weeks after each dose change	**Cough** Exclude alternative cause of cough e.g.: worsening pulmonary oedema If ACE seems likely cause consider ARB as substitute **Worsening renal function** An increase in creatinine of up to 50% above baseline or 200 µmol/l (whichever is smaller) is acceptable An increase in K^+ to ≤5.9 is acceptable Review medication list and stop any other nephrotoxic drugs if possible If K^+ rises ≥6.0 mmol/l or creatinine rises >100% or above 350 µmol/l then the ACE inhibitor should be stopped
β-Blockers Increase life expectancy Decrease hospitalization E.g.: Bisoprolol 1.25 mg od; target 10 mg od Carvedilol 3.125 mg od; target 25–50 mg bd Nebivolol 1.35 mg od*' target 10 mg od	Start at lowest dose and double the dose at not less than fortnightly intervals Monitor HR, BP and for signs of decompensation Warn patients that temporary symptomatic decompensation may occur and that overall benefit may take 3–6 months	**Worsening symptoms** Double the dose of diuretic and/or half the dose of the β-blocker. If no improvement seek specialist input. If deterioration is sudden and severe, emergency assessment may be needed **Bradycardia** ECG to exclude heart block Review medications and stop any other negative inotropes if possible **Asymptomatic low BP** No change in therapy required NB: COPD is not a contraindication to B-blockers unless there is evidence of reversible airways obstruction

Table 5.4 *(Contd.)*

Medication	Suggested dosing in the elderly	Common side effects and suggested action
Aldosterone antagonists Increase life expectancy Decrease hospitalization Eplerenone reduces mortality in patients with LV impairment post MI E.g.: Spironolactone 25 mg od Eplenerone 25 mg od	Start 25 mg od according to following criteria Spironolactone: in patients with NYHA III/IV or severe LV impairment on echo Eplerenone: in patients with heart failure post MI, or those intolerant of spironolactone Check U+Es at 1, 4, 8, and 12 weeks Late onset hyperkalaemia is sometimes seen in the elderly and diabetics so regular (3–6 monthly) monitoring of electrolytes is essential	**Deranged electrolytes** If K⁺ rises to 5.5–5.9 mmol/l or creatinine to 200 µmol/l switch to alternate day dosing and recheck If K⁺ rises ≥6.0 mmol or creatinine to >200 µmol/l (uncommon) stop drug **Gynaecomastia:** switch to eplerenone
Loop diuretics For symptomatic relief E.g.: Furosemide 20–40mg od Bumetanide 0.5–1mg od	Weigh patient Check baseline electrolytes and continue to monitor with each dose change Start at low dose: 20–40 mg od Weigh at regular intervals; uptitrate if no change. Rate of weight loss should not exceed 1 kg/24 hours A smaller maintenance dose may be needed once dry weight is reached	**Resistant oedema** In hospital a furosemide infusion over 24 hours may be tried If weight still does not respond consider adding a thiazide diuretic such as bendrofluazide or metolazone This should be done with caution and with specialist input as a large diuresis may occur causing hypotension or electrolyte imbalance

(Contd.)

Table 5.4 (Contd.)

Medication	Suggested dosing in the elderly	Common side effects and suggested action
ARBs Increase life expectancy Decrease hospitalization (similar to ACE inhibitors) E.g.: Candesartan 4 mg od; target 32 mg od	Start at lowest dose and double the dose at not less than fortnightly intervals Check U+Es at baseline and after 1–2 weeks. Recheck 1–2 weeks after each dose change **Do not co-prescribe with ACE inhibitor and aldosterone antagonist**	Generally well tolerated Do not cause cough **Worsening renal function** An increase in creatinine of up to 50% above baseline or 200 µmol/l (whichever is smaller) is acceptable. An increase in K^+ to ≤5.9 is acceptable Review medication list and stop any other nephrotoxic drugs if possible If K^+ rises ≥6.0 mmol/l or creatinine rises >100% or above 350 µmol/l then the ARB should be stopped
Digoxin Reduces hospitalization Gives symptomatic relief No evidence mortality benefit	**Indicated for:** Patients with persistent symptoms despite optimal treatment with ACE inhibitors, β-blockers and diuretics, or who are intolerant of these drugs due to hypotension Control of ventricular rate in patients with AF who are intolerant of β-blockers **Dosing:** Load with 750–1500 µg in 2 divided doses within 24 hours In an emergency, the smallest time interval permissible between loading doses is 2 hours After loading give maintenance of 62.5–250 µg depending on renal function and BMI Ensure K^+ is >4 mmol/l before initiating	**Toxicity** (Suggested by: nausea, vomiting, diarrhoea, arrhythmias, dizziness, blurred/yellow vision) Check serum level at least 6 hours post dose If symptomatic will require hospitalization for administration of 'Digibind' (digoxin specific antibody fragments)

Table 5.4 (Contd.)

Medication	Suggested dosing in the elderly	Common side effects and suggested action
Hydralazine and nitrates Decrease mortality Decrease morbidity (Mortality/morbidity effect is less than ACE inhibitors)	Consider in those who cannot tolerate ACE or ARB, especially if hypertension is a persistent **Dosing:** ISDN 20 mg tds, Hydralazine 37.5 mg tds **Target:** ISDN 40 mg tds, Hydralazine 75 mg tds	

*Indicated in patients >70 years of age based on Seniors Trial (see Chapter 11).

Additional pharmacological treatment: usual management of secondary prevention in cardiovascular disease should continue; aspirin, lipid control and good diabetic control are all important.

BMI, body mass index; COPD, chronic obstructive pulmonary disease; ISDN, isosorbide dinitrate; tds, three times daily; od, once daily; bd, twice daily; BMI, body mass index; MI, myocardial infarction; NYHA, New York Heart Association; LV, left ventricular; HR, heart rate; BP, blood pressure; U+Es, urea and electrolytes, ACE, angiotensin-converting enzyme; ARB, angiotensin receptor blocker.

Device therapy: is there a role in the elderly?

There have been great advances in pharmacological therapy for heart failure in the last decade and this is the mainstay of therapy for most patients. However, morbidity and mortality remain high and implanted medical devices are gaining increasing utility and have the potential to revolutionize the treatment of heart failure. Most of the trials to date have been in younger patients so we still await conclusive evidence that this therapy is beneficial in the elderly, but age alone should not be a contraindication (see Cardiac resynchronization therapy).

Implantable defibrillator therapy

The implantable cardioverter-defibrillator (ICD) is an important component in the management of patients with systolic left ventricular dysfunction (both ischaemic and non-ischaemic) and symptomatic chronic heart failure. Clinical trial data show a significant reduction in the overall mortality of patients with mild and moderate heart failure, but as with many heart failure trials, the elderly have not been included. (See the NICE guidelines in Box 5.3).

Cardiac resynchronization therapy (CRT)

This involves resynchronization of the failing ventricles by pacing the right and left ventricles simultaneously (also referred to as biventricular pacing). CRT with (CRT-D) or without (CRT-P) a back-up ICD, improves symptoms, quality of life, exercise tolerance, left ventricular function, and the survival of patients with advanced heart failure compared with optimal pharmacological therapy. Approximately 30% of patients do not respond and the reasons for this remain unclear. Limited trial evidence exists in the elderly but in one observational study of 266 patients undergoing CRT, 107 were >75 years and experienced improvements in clinical and echocardiographic parameters comparable with younger participants.

The NICE recommendations for CRT are shown in Box 5.3 and should be followed in the elderly if they otherwise have a reasonable expectation of survival with good functional status of over 1 year. With increasing expertise and evidence these indications may change in the future.

Box 5.3 NICE guidelines for CRT (TA120, 2007) and ICD (TA95, 2006)

CRT with a pacing device (CRT-P) is recommended as a treatment option for people with heart failure who fulfil all the following criteria:
- NYHA class III–IV symptoms
- Receiving optimal therapy
- In sinus rhythm either with:
  - QRS duration of >150 ms or QRS duration of 120–149 ms and mechanical dyssynchrony confirmed by echocardiography
  - LVEF ≤35%.

CRT with a defibrillator device (CRT-D) may be considered for people who fulfil the criteria for implantation of a CRT-P device above and who separately fulfil the criteria for the use of an ICD device as recommended in NICE TA95.

For secondary prevention ICDs are recommended for patients who present, in the absence of a treatable cause, with one of the following:
- Survived a cardiac arrest due to ventricular tachycardia (VT) or ventricular fibrillation
- Spontaneous sustained VT causing syncope or significant haemodynamic compromise
- Sustained VT without syncope or cardiac arrest, with ejection fraction <35%.

For primary prevention, ICDs are recommended for patients with a history of previous (more than 4 weeks) myocardial infarction and either:
- Left ventricular dysfunction with an LVEF of less than 35% and non-sustained VT on Holter (24-hour ECG) monitoring and inducible VT on electrophysiological testing or
- Left ventricular dysfunction with an LVEF of less than 30% and QRS duration of ≥120 ms

Important points to remember when considering ICD and/ or CRT in the elderly

- Quality rather than quantity of life is more important to most elderly patients.
- The risk of procedure complications is likely to be higher due to problems with vascular access and increased risk of infection etc.
- CRT-D devices may deliver inappropriate defibrillating shocks, which may be distressing for patients and impair their quality of life.
- Patients with ICD and or CRT require regular clinic follow-up which some elderly patients may find difficult or interferes significantly with their quality of life.
- Timing and appropriateness of switching off the defibrillator device need to be addressed as end of life approaches and the patient is in the palliative stage.

Device therapy in the future

A number of devices are approved or under development to monitor heart failure, ranging from interactive weight scales to implantable continuous pressure monitors. We still await conclusive evidence that this technology can improve patient outcomes but it may prove especially useful in the elderly.

Heart replacement with left ventricular assist devices has been evaluated for several decades. At present mechanical devices in the UK are only available in specialized centers with limited indications such as a bridge to transplantation or in those with a reversible cause for heart failure, such as acute myocarditis, and are not at present applicable to the elderly.

Mechanical methods of remodelling the heart have been under investigation for several years but most of the earlier methods have not proved useful in the longer term. New methods of restraining the heart with prosthetic material are under investigation in humans, with encouraging pilot results.

Surgical treatment for heart failure

- As yet there are no randomized controlled trials for revascularization in patients who present with heart failure, so this is at present only recommended as for ischaemia (Chapter 2), particularly in the elderly, who have a higher operative mortality and morbidity.
- Surgery for patients with valve lesions is discussed in Chapter 3.
- Cardiomyoplasty is no longer recommended.

Specific treatment issues in the elderly

Polypharmacy

- Elderly patients in heart failure inevitably have many tablets to take.
- Medication should be reviewed every 6 months and rationalized.
- Dosset boxes/blister packs are useful for those with cognitive impairment.
- If concordance is still poor, explore this with the patient e.g.: if diuresis is causing a problem could the timing of furosemide be altered?
- Check if side effects are an issue and consider altering drugs if necessary, e.g.: try an ARB if the ACE inhibitor is causing an irritating cough.

Cognitive impairment

As patient education is the key to good concordance with therapy, cognitively impaired patients pose a particular problem. Remember that emphasis should be placed on quality of life; if only a few tablets are being taken each day, focus on the ones that bring symptomatic relief. In addition heart failure may lead to worsening of any pre-existing cognitive impairment and this should be explained to carers and families.

If the patient is able, take time in a non-crisis setting (e.g.: heart failure nurse clinic, general practice) to explore advance care planning (Chapter 13), should the patient's medical condition acutely deteriorate. This is true for all patients with heart failure, but especially important for those who may lose capacity over time.

Renal impairment

In heart failure patients renal dysfunction is linked to increased morbidity and mortality. Many drugs used for the treatment of heart failure are potentially nephrotoxic. A balance has to be accepted which will usually involve a slight deterioration in renal function and a small amount of remaining oedema.

Approach

- Review the diagnosis: what is the cause of renal impairment and can it be improved?
- Review medications: is the patient on any other nephrotoxic drugs and can they be downtitrated or stopped?
- Start new medication at a low dose and uptitrate slowly.
- In cases of extreme diuretic resistant fluid overload plus renal failure, ultrafiltration may be an option. The evidence base for this is currently limited and it is unlikely to be appropriate in a frail elderly patient.
- If treatment is commenced in hospital, complete medication changes and concurrent monitoring of weight and electrolytes before discharge.
- Only discharge earlier if the patient will be monitored closely at home by a heart failure nurse.

Coexistent chronic obstructive pulmonary disease (COPD)

Patients with congestive cardiac failure (CCF) may have coexistent COPD. This can lead to difficulties in diagnosis as they present with similar symptoms and signs so a low threshold of suspicion is essential to avoid missing heart failure in this patient group. Cor pulmonale is right heart failure secondary to pulmonary disease. This is a separate entity which can cause confusion in the diagnosis and is discussed later in this chapter. Treatment of heart failure in COPD patients should follow the guidelines as above. There is concern about using β-blockers in patients with COPD, but in the absence of reversible airways obstruction, they should be prescribed as there is evidence of mortality benefit in COPD patients treated with β-blockers.

Acute heart failure

Treatment of acute heart failure in the elderly is identical to that in younger patients. Acute presentation may be the first presentation of heart failure. However, those with known chronic heart failure may decompensate as a result of cardiac ischaemia, poor medication compliance, infection, or tachyarrhythmia such as AF. In the elderly, a combination of all four is not uncommon.

The classic patient with acute heart failure will be wheeled into the emergency room in the early hours of the morning. They will be pale, clammy, and gasping for breath – often grabbing the sides of the trolley and leaning forwards to try to increase their tidal volume. They may be hypoxic and agitated. Patients liken it to breathing with a plastic bag over their head. Swift action is needed and the patient should be stabilized in the resuscitation area.

Diagnosis

In this circumstance history taking will be limited, although accompanying family members may help.

Examine the patient for signs of fluid overload and for clues as to why they have decompensated.

- Tachycardia and tachypnoea.
- Raised JVP.
- Crackles in the lung fields and pleural effusions.
- Oedema in the legs and sacrum.
- Do they have an infection: look for a temperature, productive cough, or signs of consolidation in the chest.
- Do they have an arrhythmia or cardiac ischaemia: feel the pulse and do an ECG.
- Remember to consider alternative diagnoses to heart failure.
- Remember troponin may be elevated in heart failure itself and is a bad prognostic sign. It does not always indicate acute coronary syndrome (ACS). It is important to be aware of this and avoid unnecessary treatment especially as aspirin may interfere with action of ACE (see Table 5.3).
- Check NT-proBNP if available as studies have shown that this can help distinguish respiratory and cardiac causes of acute dyspnoea in the emergency setting.

Initial management

While examining the patient ask a colleague to:

- Attach high-flow oxygen (but not if COPD is present; remember it may coexist)
- Attach the patient to a monitor and check their blood pressure and oxygen saturations
- Gain intravenous access and take bloods (full blood count, urea and electrolytes, liver function tests troponin, and blood cultures may be indicated)
- Perform an arterial blood gas (ABG).

Further management

If you are unsure of the diagnosis following initial assessment and the patient is stable, wait for a CXR to confirm.

If you are confident of your diagnosis **or** if the patient is unstable **do not wait** for further investigation results.

Immediate drug therapy

- Intravenous furosemide 40 mg stat. Higher doses may be needed in those on long-term high-dose oral diuretics or in renal impairment.
- Follow with opiates plus antiemetic.
- If not responding to furosemide, start a nitrate infusion if blood pressure >100 mm Hg systolic.
- Treat any underlying cause e.g.: antibiotics for infection, β-blocker or digoxin for AF (see Chapter 7, Table 7.3, p. 155).
- In patients not responding to bolus doses of furosemide start a furosemide infusion. Consider this approach early especially in patients with hypotension ± renal impairment.
- If no improvement and the patient is still struggling to ventilate, consider appropriateness of higher level care and involve the critical care team. Continuous positive airway pressure (CPAP) is a non-invasive option in the short term and is well tolerated in many elderly patients so age should not be a contraindication.
- Once stabilized review existing therapy and optimize or initiate investigation and treatment as for chronic heart failure if this is a new diagnosis.

Palliative care for heart failure

End-stage heart failure is increasingly being managed in the community by palliative care teams as their non-cancer services expand. A multidisciplinary structured programme of care is needed.

Timing of referral is complex as it is difficult to predict when a patient is likely to deteriorate for the last time. Advance care planning should be encouraged; although these conversations are difficult they will greatly improve the end-of-life experience for the patient and increase the chances of them dying in their preferred place of care.

Management should focus entirely on symptom control. This may include opiates (e.g.: liquid morphine) to relieve symptoms of breathlessness and this can be especially helpful at night. Palliative oxygen can also be supplied at home. Medication should be reviewed regularly and withdrawing and adjusting doses should not only be in response to adverse effects. The priority is to continue drugs given for symptom control versus those for prognostic benefit.

Patients and family and carers education about the goals of palliative treatment and role of pacemakers and ICDs should help relieve anxiety at the end of life. Discussion should include the issue of switching off the defibrillator component of the device. Ideally this should be addressed at the time of implantation and reviewed regularly thereafter. Sudden arrhythmic death may be preferable to some patients with end-stage heart failure rather than the alternative of progressive symptom deterioration.

The Liverpool Care of the Dying pathway is increasingly used in end-of-life care in all specialities. It has not been studied specifically in heart failure but from personal experience it can be very useful in this group of patients.

Cor pulmonale

- Cor pulmonale is the impairment in right ventricular function as a result of respiratory disease.
- Chronic hypoxia leading to pulmonary arteriolar constriction and pulmonary hypertension is the principal pathophysiological mechanism.
- It is usually a chronic, progressive process, but can occur acutely due to sudden increase in pulmonary artery pressure as in pulmonary embolism or acute exacerbation of COPD.
- It is a separate entity from heart failure due to left ventricular dysfunction but can present similarly, so careful assessment and investigation are essential to avoid misdiagnosis and unnecessary treatment.

Causes

- The commonest cause is chronic obstructive pulmonary disease (COPD).
- Other causes include:
  - Parenchymal lung disease, e.g. pulmonary fibrosis
  - Neuromuscular disorders causing chronic hypoventilation, e.g. motor neuron disease
  - Obstructive or central sleep apnoea
  - Thoracic deformity, e.g. kyphoscoliosis
  - Recurrent pulmonary emboli.

Symptoms

Common symptoms of cor pulmonale include:
- Tachypnoea (particularly at rest) and exertional dyspnoea
- Fatigue and lassitude
- Ankle swelling
- Angina-type chest discomfort – often non-responsive to nitrates (thought to be due to right ventricular ischaemia)
- Haemoptysis (due to pulmonary arteriolar rupture)
- Hepatic congestion in late stage (anorexia, jaundice, and right upper quadrant abdominal discomfort).

Signs

- Cyanosis and plethora.
- Hyper-expanded chest, decreased air entry, crackles and wheeze in chest due to underlying pulmonary disease.
- Left parasternal heave (sign of right ventricular hypertrophy).
- Distended neck veins with raised JVP and visible a or v waves and hepatojugular reflux.
- Peripheral oedema (pitting).
- 3rd/4th heart sounds and pan-systolic murmur of tricuspid regurgitation over right heart.
- Split second heart sound with loud pulmonary component.
- Diastolic pulmonary regurgitation murmur over pulmonary artery (advanced sign).
- Hepatomegaly ± pulsatile liver if significant tricuspid regurgitation.
- Ascites (advanced sign).

Differential diagnosis in the elderly
- Congestive cardiac failure due to primary cardiac disease.
- Right-sided heart failure due to right-ventricular myocardial infarction.
- Late presentation of untreated atrial or ventricular septal defect.

Investigation of underlying cardiopulmonary disease in the elderly
Investigations may be needed to determine the cause(s) of respiratory disease leading to cor pulmonale
- CXR (Fig. 5.5)
- Spirometry/pulmonary function tests including gas transfer and flow volume loop
- Computed tomography (CT)/magnetic resonance imaging (MRI) of the chest
- Ventilation/perfusion scan/spiral-CT angiography (if acute or recurrent pulmonary embolism suspected).

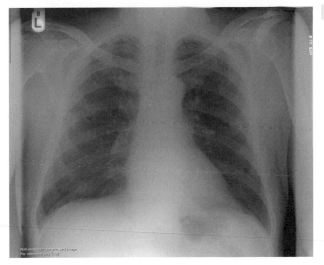

Fig. 5.5 CXR showing hyperinflated lungs and normal heart size in a patient with severe emphysema and cor pulmonale but good left ventricular systolic function on echocardiogram.

Investigation of right heart function and cardiopulmonary function
- ECG (evidence of right ventricular hypertrophy (Fig. 5.6)/arrhythmias such as AF).
- Full blood count to determine haematocrit if there is secondary polycythaemia.
- ABG on room air and in response to administration of oxygen.
- Measure NT-proBNP if available (elevated BNP levels have been shown to correlate with raised pulmonary artery pressures and cor pulmonale).
- Echocardiography and Doppler – for assessment of right ventricular size and function and estimation of pulmonary artery systolic pressure.
- Other available tests include thoracic MRI, radionuclide ventriculography, and right heart catheterization are rarely indicated in the elderly as they add little to management at present.

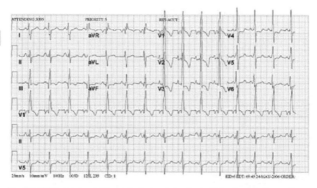

Fig. 5.6 ECG showing right ventricular hypertrophy and 'p' pulmonale in a patient with cor pulmonale and clinical evidence of pulmonary hypertension.

Management

Acute cor pulmonale is treated by correcting the underlying precipitant usually acute pulmonary embolism or an infective exacerbation of COPD.

Chronic cor pulmonale involves treatment of the underlying cause and specific treatment

- Long-term oxygen therapy (LTOT) improves quality of life and survival in patients with severe chronic hypoxia due to lung disease, by reducing pulmonary arteriolar constriction and improving/slowing the progression of cor pulmonale. It is recommended if PaO_2 <7.3 kPa or between 7.3kPa and 8 kPa and there is another risk factor (haematocrit >55%, nocturnal hypoxia, pulmonary hypertension, peripheral oedema). It must be used for 15 hours/day to be effective. There are recent guidelines from the British Thoracic Society on oxygen therapy (www.brit-thoracic.org.uk/).
- Diuretics such as furosemide and bumetanide are useful if right ventricular filling volume is elevated with associated peripheral oedema. Avoid over-diuresis, which can impair the function of both ventricles. Take care to maintain K^+ as a hypokalaemic metabolic alkalosis can reduce respiratory drive through reducing the hypercapnic stimulus to breathe. Intravenous diuretics may be required in acute decompensation, due to poor absorption of medication from the oedematous gut. Bumetanide may be preferable to furosemide as oral therapy, as it is better absorbed.
- Digoxin is sometimes used but there is little evidence for efficacy. It may he useful to control ventricular rate in AF if β-blockers or rate-slowing calcium antagonists are not tolerated.
- Methylxanthine bronchodilators such as theophylline are used for their beneficial effect on bronchial tone and have a mild positive inotropic effect but there is little evidence for their efficacy.
- In patients in whom venous thromboembolism is the underlying cause, anticoagulation with warfarin is indicated.
- Venesection may be required in severe secondary polycythaemia (haematocrit >0.65) but should be used with caution. It may improve symptoms but there is no evidence of improved survival.

Prognosis

This depends on the underlying cause and its rate of progression. The 2-year mortality for cor pulmonale complicating COPD is high, particularly for those who continue to smoke. The 5-year mortality is around 60%, even in treated patients. Disease progression can be slowed and prognosis significantly improved by smoking cessation and appropriate use of LTOT.

Guidelines and references

Hunt SA, Abraham WT, Chin MH, Feldman AM, Francis GS, Ganiats TG, *et al.*; American College of Cardiology Foundation; American Heart Association (2009) 2009 Focused update incorporated into the ACC/AHA 2005 Guidelines for the Diagnosis and Management of Heart Failure in Adults A Report of the American College of Cardiology Foundation/American Heart Association Task Force on Practice Guidelines Developed in Collaboration With the International Society for Heart and Lung Transplantation. *Circulation* **119**:391–479. Available from: www.americanheart.org.

National Institute for Health and Clinical Excellence (2003, currently being updated) Management of chronic heart failure in adults in primary and secondary care. Clinical guideline 5. London: National Institute for Health and Clinical Excellence. Available from: www.nice.org.uk/CG005.

National Institute for Health and Clinical Excellence (2006) Implantable cardioverter defibrillators for arrhythmias. Technology appraisal 95. London: National Institute for Health and Clinical Excellence. Available from: www.nice.org.uk/TA095.

National Institute for Health and Clinical Excellence (2006) Short-term circulatory support with left ventricular assist devices as a bridge to cardiac transplantation or recovery. Interventional procedure 177. London: National Institute for Health and Clinical Excellence. Available from: www.nice.org.uk/IPG177.

National Institute for Health and Clinical Excellence (2007) Cardiac resynchronisation therapy for the treatment of heart failure. Technology Appraisal 120. London: National Institute for Health and Clinical Excellence. Available from: www.nice.org.uk/TA120.

Scottish Intercollegiate Guidelines Network (2007) Management of chronic heart failure. SIGN guideline 95. Edinburgh: Scottish Intercollegiate Guidelines Network. Available at: www.sign.ac.uk.

Task Force for Diagnosis and Treatment of Acute and Chronic Heart Failure 2008 of European Society of Cardiology, Dickstein K, Cohen-Solal A, Filippatos G, McMurray JJ, Ponikowski P, Poole-Wilson PA, *et al.* (2008) ESC Guidelines for the diagnosis and treatment of acute and chronic heart failure 2008: the Task Force for the Diagnosis and Treatment of Acute and Chronic Heart Failure 2008 of the European Society of Cardiology. Developed in collaboration with the Heart Failure Association of the ESC (HFA) and endorsed by the European Society of Intensive Care Medicine (ESICM). *Eur Heart J* **29**:2388–42. Available at: www.escardio.org.

Chapter 6

Arrhythmias in the elderly

Arrhythmias in the elderly

- Arrhythmias are a significant cause of morbidity and mortality in the elderly.
- Arrhythmias result mainly from age-related changes and hypertension, coronary artery disease, systolic and diastolic heart failure, and valve disease.
- Patients may be asymptomatic or have symptoms ranging from non-specific to paroxysms of palpitations, to syncope and may present with sudden cardiac death.

Atrial fibrillation is the commonest arrhythmia in the elderly and is discussed in Chapter 7. Other arrhythmias are listed in Table 6.1, and those relevant to the elderly will be discussed in more detail here.

Table 6.1 Cardiac arrhythmias in the elderly

Bradyarrhythmia

- Sinus node dysfunction
- Sinus bradycardia
- Sinus arrest
- Sick sinus syndrome/brady-tachy syndrome
- Atrioventricular conduction defect
- Type I second degree AV block (Mobitz I or Wenckebach)
- Type II second degree AV block (Mobitz II)
- Complete heart block

Tachyarrhythmia

- Supraventricular tachyarrhythmia
  - Atrioventricular nodal node re-entrant tachycardia (AVNRT)
  - Atrioventricular tachycardia with WPW (AVRT) – rare in elderly
  - Atrial tachycardia
  - Atrial flutter
  - Atrial fibrillation
- Ventricular tachycardia
  - Monomorphic ventricular tachycardia
  - Polymorphic ventricular tachycardia
  - Ventricular fibrillation

Arrhythmias due to pacemaker malfunction

- Bradycardia due to:
  - Battery or generator failure
  - Electrode dysfunction
  - Interference (myopotential or electromagnetic)
  - Inappropriate programming
- Pacemaker-mediated tachycardia
- Pacemaker syndrome

The cardiac conduction system and age

- With normal ageing there is fibrosis and calcification of the atrioventricular (AV) node and bundle branches, and an increase in fibrosis and loss of myocardial fibres in the sinoatrial (SA) node.
- This leads to sinus node dysfunction and AV block.
- Amyloid deposition may also be important.

Bradyarrhythmias

Sinus node dysfunction

- The prevalence of sinus node dysfunction increases with age.
- It may manifest as sinus bradycardia, sinus arrest, or brady-tachy (sick sinus (SSS)) syndrome.
- The commonest cause is fibrosis of the SA node and loss of pacemaker cells with age.
- Secondary causes to exclude are listed in Box 6.1.
- In addition to SA node dysfunction there is atrial abnormality, which is the substrate for the development of atrial tachyarrhythmias.

Box 6.1 Secondary causes of sinus node dysfunction and AV block

- Drugs:
  - Most common: β-blockers, non-dihydropyridine calcium channel antagonists (rate slowing), digoxin, amiodarone, class 1 anti-arrhythmic drugs, anticholinesterase inhibitors (rare, see Chapter 14)
- Hypothyroidism
- Hypothermia
- Electrolyte disturbances (hyperkalaemia)
- Infiltrative disorders such as amyloid, sarcoid, and haemachromatosis

---

- *Sinus bradycardia*: Heart rates of 35–40 beats/min do not usually reduce cerebral perfusion sufficiently to cause symptoms in normal individuals. However, elderly patients with associated cardiovascular and cerebrovascular disease may have symptoms such as presyncope, fatigue, and dyspnoea. Whether slow heart rates contribute to cognitive impairment is still debated but rates consistently less than 40 bpm may be a factor in some patients.
- *Sinus pauses* of <3 seconds are not usually associated with symptoms, whereas those ≥3 seconds may cause syncope or presyncope. In the absence of symptoms, be cautious in interpreting sinus arrest as a cause of syncope.
- *SSS (Brady-tachy syndrome)* is characterized by bouts of sinus bradycardia, sinus pauses and episodes of atrial tachyarrhythmia. Symptoms include palpitations, syncope, presyncope, fatigue, and weakness.
- *Chronotropic incompetence* is characterized by impaired heart rate response to exercise (usually <85% of age predicted maximum) and typically presents with reduced exercise tolerance.

Diagnosis and investigation

- ECGs are typically normal if asymptomatic at the time.
- Ambulatory 24-hour tapes can be diagnostic.
- Event recorders and longer periods of monitoring may be helpful if symptoms are infrequent.

- An implantable reveal device (see Chapter 8) may be required for diagnosis if initial investigations are negative and there is a high index of suspicion.
- Blood tests are required to exclude reversible causes (thyroid-stimulating hormone (TSH), renal function, and electrolytes).

Management

- Remove precipitating cause if possible. However, this may not be possible if there is an absolute indication to continue treatment e.g. β-blockers to control tachyarrhythmias in SSS.
- Permanent pacing (see Permanent pacemakers, p. 130): SA node dysfunction (bradycardia) with symptoms is an absolute indication for permanent pacemaker insertion. Tachycardias often follow on bradycardias so pacemaker insertion may also reduce tachyarrhythmias.

AV (heart) block

- Heart block is a common cause of dizziness and syncope in the elderly.
- It may be transient and infrequent and therefore, difficult to demonstrate.
- The clinical significance depends on the site and the degree of the block.
- Age-related fibrosis is the most common cause in the Western world.
- Other causes of heart block are listed in Box 6.1, with the addition of acute myocardial infarction and calcific aortic stenosis.

1st degree AV nodal block

This is the most common AV nodal block in the elderly. Each atrial beat is conducted to the ventricle, however, the impulse conduction is slowed through the AV node. It is usually asymptomatic and does not require treatment.

Diagnosis

The electrocardiogram (ECG) shows prolonged PR interval (>200ms).

2nd degree AV block (Mobitz type I and II)

Mobitz type I, also known as Wenckebach, shows progressively slowed conduction through the AV node before eventually an atrial beat is not conducted to the ventricles. It is usually asymptomatic and not an indication for pacing on its own.

Mobitz type II shows fixed conduction through the AV node and atrial beats are not conducted to the ventricles at regular and predictable intervals. Mobitz type II block has a high risk of progressing to complete heart block. Patients may be asymptomatic or present with syncope and presyncope, or with dyspnoea, fatigue, or evidence of heart failure.

Diagnosis
- Mobitz type I – ECG shows progressive lengthening of the PR interval before eventually a complex is dropped and the circuit restarts.
- Mobitz type II – ECG shows fixed PR interval but complexes are lost at regular intervals giving rise to so called 2:1, 3:1 block (Fig. 6.1 shows 2:1 block).

Investigations – as outlined for sinus node dysfunction above.

Management – exclude reversible causes (Box 6.1): Mobitz type II block has the potential to progress to complete heart block and is an indication for permanent pacemaker insertion.

3rd degree (complete) heart block (CHB)
In this type of block no beats are conducted between the atria and the ventricles. Often the atria and the ventricles beat regularly but at completely different rates and not in synchronicity with each other. Be suspicious of this rhythm when the pulse is <40 bpm. It is usually due to fibrosis of the conduction system but can occur in acute myocardial infarction especially an inferior infarct. Patients may be asymptomatic or present with syncope and presyncope, or with dyspnoea, fatigue, or evidence of heart failure.

Diagnosis
The ECG typically shows bradycardia with a rate of <40 bpm and no correlation between the p waves and the QRS complexes (see Fig. 6.2). It may be intermittent so investigation as for sinus node dysfunction may be required. Check troponin to exclude myocardial infarction if onset is acute.

Management
- Exclude reversible causes (Box 6.1), including acute myocardial infarction.
- Referral for permanent pacemaker (even if asymptomatic as increased risk of sudden death).
- If caused by inferior myocardial infarction it is usually transient and does not affect prognosis so permanent pacing is not usually required unless it persists. In anterior myocardial infarction the development of CHB indicates extensive infarction and pacing and implantation of an implantable cardioverter-defibrillator (ICD) is usually recommended.

Bundle branch block (BBB)
- Common in the elderly (17% over age 80).
- **Bifascicular block** is the combination of right BBB (RBBB) and left anterior fascicle block (Fig. 6.3).
- **Trifascicular block** is a misnomer and is the combination of 1st degree heart block and bifascicular block.

The risk of progression to complete heart block is low (approx 1% per year) so asymptomatic bifascicular and trifascicular blocks are not an indication for permanent pacing.

Patients who have intermittent symptomatic AV block (Mobitz type II or complete) require permanent pacing.

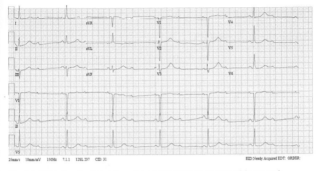

Fig. 6.1 ECG showing 2:1 atrioventricular block in an 80-year-old man with presyncope.

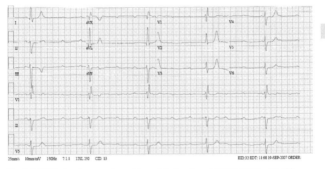

Fig. 6.2 ECG showing complete atrioventricular dissociation in an 88-year-old woman presenting with collapse.

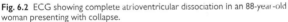

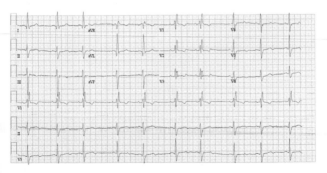

Fig. 6.3 ECG showing bifascicular block: right bundle branch block and left axis deviation with sinus rhythm in asymptomatic 78-year-old man.

Pacemakers

Temporary pacemakers

- Transvenous temporary cardiac pacing is a potentially life-saving procedure in patients with asystole and heart block associated with syncope and hypotension.
- Unfortunately in inexperienced hands it is associated with a high complication rate – related to complications of central venous access, wire positioning, and infection.
- Outside of cardiac centres, unless there is local expertise, it is usually best to stabilize the patient using external pacing or isoprenaline infusion and transfer to the nearest cardiac centre for temporary or permanent pacing as soon as possible.
- Transvenous pacing may be required to cover non-cardiac surgical procedures due to persistent or intermittent CHB or Mobitz type II block, and should be performed by a person experienced in the procedure. It is often better to delay non-essential surgery until a permanent system is inserted.
- Overdrive pacing may occasionally be useful in recurrent tachyarrhythmias such as torsades de pointes (see Ventricular tachycardia, p. 140).

Permanent pacemakers

The terminology used to describe permanent pacemakers applies to the chamber paced, the chamber sensed, the response to sensing, and the programmable capability as shown in Box 6.2. The type of device inserted depends largely on the indication, and functional capacity of the individual and for most elderly patients will either be a single or dual chamber device with (Fig. 6.4) or without rate responsive mode.

Box 6.3 summarizes the National Institute for Health and Clinical Excellence (NICE) guidelines for pacing in SSS and AV block. NICE recommends physiological pacing in most patients but the evidence base for this is still unclear and single chamber ventricular pacing may be equally beneficial in the elderly (see Chapter 11).

Box 6.2 Pacemaker nomenclature

- The first letter of the code signifies the chamber being paced:
A = atrium, V = ventricle, D= dual = A+V
- The second letter signifies the chamber being sensed:
A = atrium, V = ventricle, D= dual = A+V
- The third letter signifies the response to sensing:
I = inhibited, T = triggered, D = dual = T+I
- The fourth letter signifies rate modulation:
O (or no letter) = none, R = rate modulation
- The fifth letter signifies multi-site pacing:
O (or no letter) = none, A = atrium, V = ventricle, D = dual (A+V)

E.g. DDDR refers to a dual chamber pacemaker with rate modulation.

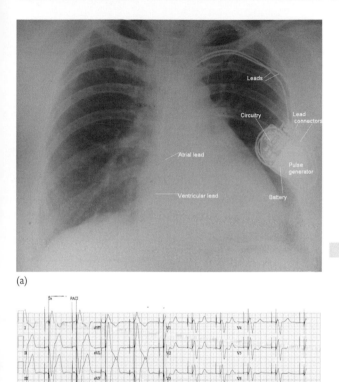

(a)

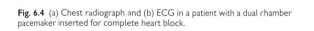

(b)

Fig. 6.4 (a) Chest radiograph and (b) ECG in a patient with a dual chamber pacemaker inserted for complete heart block.

Box 6.3 NICE guidelines for pacing for symptomatic bradycardia in SSS and/or AV block (NICE 2005)

Dual chamber pacing is recommended for all patients except:
- Patients with SSS and intact AV conduction where single chamber atrial pacing may be appropriate. This is rarely the case in the elderly.
- AV block in patients with persistent atrial fibrillation where single chamber ventricular pacing is recommended.
- Patient specific factors such as frailty, co-morbidities, etc., influence the balance of risk in favour of single chamber ventricular pacing.

Complications of pacemaker insertion
These may be divided into early and late.

Common early complications
These include:
- Intraoperative pneumothorax and haemothorax
- Haematoma
- Infection
- Lead dislodgement (especially the atrial lead).

Late complications
- *Pacemaker syndrome.* This refers to a group of symptoms including nausea, palpitations, chest pain, fatigue, breathlessness, presyncope, and syncope. It is thought to be caused by loss of the heart's natural AV sequence in single chamber ventricular pacing. Difficulties in diagnosis arise due to overlap with symptoms of cardiac disease, and with symptoms arising from co-morbidities. Severe symptoms may require upgrade to a dual chamber pacemaker.
- *Pacemaker dysfunction as a result of electromagnetic interference.* The use of electrocautery, lithotripsy, radiofrequency ablation, and magnetic resonance imaging (MRI), can lead to pacemaker malfunction so reprogramming and monitoring are important. Clinical significant interference is rare from the use of cell phones provided they are held more than 15 cm from the pacemaker, and with electronic surveillance equipment in libraries and airports provided the patient passes through quickly.
- *Pacemaker mediated tachycardia* can usually be addressed by reprogramming of the device.
- *Device failure* will usually be picked up by regular monitoring of the device to detect approaching end-of-life parameters but can occasionally arise without warning as a result of interference or lead dislodgement or fracture. Pacemaker function should be checked in patients presenting with presyncope or syncope.

Tachyarrhythmias

Tachyarrhythmias are often subdivided into narrow QRS complex and wide QRS complex arrhythmias. Narrow complex arise in the atria or AV node and are referred to as supraventricular (SVT) and wide complex usually arise in the ventricles (VT) but can occasionally be due to an SVT with bundle branch block or aberrant conduction.

Supraventricular tachyarrhythmias

The causes, ECG diagnosis, response to adenosine, and management options for SVTs in the elderly are summarized in Table 6.2. Patients may present typically with palpitation but atypical presentations with dyspnoea, chest pain, weakness, syncope, and presyncope are more frequent than in younger patients. Non-sustained SVTs are not infrequently found during 24-hour ECG monitoring in the elderly, and in the absence of symptoms rarely require treatment. *If the patient is haemodynamically compromised immediate DC cardioversion and resuscitation are essential.*

Vagal manoeuvres and adenosine in SVTs

Vagal manoeuvres can be used to terminate SVTs but are generally less effective in the elderly. Carotid sinus stimulation should be avoided in those with carotid bruits and or cerebrovascular disease because of the risk of embolization. Adenosine is the first-line pharmacological treatment if the patient is haemodynamically stable. It has a short half-life and is effective, but it cannot be used in patients with asthma and may precipitate ventricular fibrillation in patients with coronary artery disease.

Table 6.2 Supraventricular arrhythmias

Rhythm	ECG diagnosis	Causes and risk factors	Response to adenosine	Management
Sinus tachycardia (ST)	Sinus rhythm Rate >100 bpm	Physiological (stress, emotion, pain) Pathological (heart failure, hypovolaemia, hypoxia, hyperthyroidism) Drugs (caffeine, amphetamine, β agonists)	No response	Look for and treat the underlying cause
Atrial tachycardia (AT)	Regular tachycardia between 130 and 200 bpm P wave morphology different from sinus rhythm 1:1 conduction usually	Usually an ectopic atrial focus May be caused by digoxin toxicity Usually paroxysmal	No response	Correct electrolytes Check digoxin levels if indicated β-blocker or rate-slowing calcium channel antagonist to slow ventricular rate may be required if rhythm persists or patient is compromised
Multifocal atrial tachycardia (MAT)	Irregular tachycardia with ≥3 different P wave morphologies Often misdiagnosed as atrial fibrillation	Usually seen in elderly patients with chronic obstructive pulmonary disease (COPD)	No response	Treat underlying condition Correct electrolyte abnormalities

(Contd.)

Table 6.2 (*Contd.*)

Rhythm	ECG diagnosis	Causes and risk factors	Response to adenosine	Management
Atrial flutter	ECG shows rapid atrial contraction (p wave rate ~300) with absence of flat baseline between beats (Fig. 6.5) usually regular but may be irregular if there is variable AV block	Results from macro-re-entrant circuit in either the right (most common) or left atrium with a typical atrial rate of 250–350 Risk factors include: Age (100 times more common in those over 80 than in young patients) COPD Heart failure	Increase atrio-ventricular (AV) block so that flutter waves become more apparent transiently	Treat underlying condition Correct electrolyte abnormalities Increased thrombo-embolic risk so requires anticoagulation as discussed for atrial fibrillation in Chapter 7 Rate control* Electrical cardioversion† Pharmacological cardioversion‡ Radiofrequency ablation or AV nodal ablation and pacing§
Atrio-ventricular nodal re-entrant tachycardia (AVNRT)	Regular narrow complex tachycardia with no discernable P waves before the QRS complex. P waves may be detected in or after the QRS complex (Fig. 6.6)	Re-entrant circuit within the AV node Usually paroxysmal	Terminates arrhythmia in 90%	Correct electrolytes Electrical cardioversion in acute episodes if adenosine fails or patient is haemodynamically compromised. Pharmacological therapy with β-blockers and rate limiting Calcium channel antagonists to prevent paroxysms Sotalol or amiodarone as second line Pill in the pocket¶ Radiofrequency ablation**

Table 6.2 (Contd.)

Rhythm	ECG diagnosis	Causes and risk factors	Response to adenosine	Management
Atrio-ventricular re-entrant tachycardia (AVRT)	Narrow complex tachycardia with no discernable P waves before the QRS complex. If antegrade conduction is across the accessory (fast) pathway the QRS complex will be broad. ECG between paroxysms may reveal pre-excitation with short PR interval ± slurred QRS upstroke	Re-entrant circuit is extranodal e.g. Wolff Parkinson White (WPW) Rare in elderly Usually paroxysmal	Terminates regular narrow complex tachycardia in 90% Avoid if the rhythm is irregular and/or broad complex	Electrical cardioversion is the preferred treatment acutely especially if QRS is broad Avoid drugs that slow AV node conduction Radiofrequency ablation is the treatment of choice due to risk of ventricular fibrillation and sudden death

*Rate control** is the option for most patients. B-blockers, non-dihydropyridine calcium channel antagonists (verapamil and diltiazem), and digoxin can all be effective either alone or in combination as discussed for atrial fibrillation in Chapter 7. High doses may be required and therefore side effects are common. Remember diltiazem increases serum digoxin levels so monitoring is important.

†Atrial flutter is very sensitive to **DC cardioversion**, which can be achieved with low voltages (50–150 V). Recurrence rates are high so this is reserved for elderly patients who remain symptomatic or are intolerant of rate-control treatment.

‡**Pharmacological cardioversion**. Atrial flutter is relatively insensitive. Amiodarone is the only available agent in the UK as class IC agents such as flecainide are contraindicated in the elderly because of structural or ischaemic heart disease. If flecainide is used it should be used in combination with a B-blocker or rate-slowing calcium channel antagonist due to the risk of 1:1 AV conduction.

§**Radiofrequency ablation** is the most effective way of treating atrial flutter and maintaining sinus rhythm. It is invasive and experience in the elderly is limited so the success rate and complication rate in this age group are unknown. It is usually reserved for patients who remain symptomatic in spite of more conservative treatment and who are otherwise reasonably fit and active. These patients should be referred to an arrhythmia specialist for further assessment. **AV node ablation and pacing** is an alternative option in some patients.

¶**'Pill in the pocket'** approach may be considered in those with infrequent symptoms. The combination of diltiazem 120 mg and propranolol 80 mg is most effective but beware of using in the elderly due to risk of bradycardia and hypotension.

**Radiofrequency ablation is now considered the most effective curative treatment for AVNRT but experience in the elderly is limited. Complications are higher due to friable cardiac structures more prone to catheter perforation, associated cardiovascular co-morbidities, increased risk of atrial fibrillation and thrombo-embolism, and difficult cardiovascular access. Patients with frequent symptoms not responding to or intolerant of pharmacological therapy should be referred to an arrhythmia specialist for assessment.

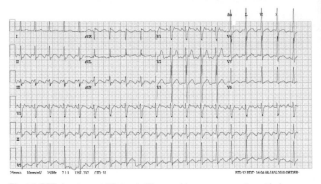

Fig. 6.5 ECG showing atrial flutter in 82-year-old woman presenting with dyspnoea. The characteristic negative atrial waves in the inferior leads are seen (saw tooth morphology).

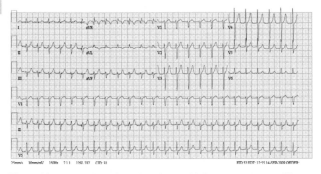

Fig. 6.6 Narrow complex tachycardia with no visible P waves in a 72-year-old man presenting with palpitation and syncope. Cardioverted to sinus rhythm with intravenous adenosine.

Ventricular tachycardia

- Sustained *monomophic ventricular tachycardia (VT)* is seen in patients with organic heart disease, most commonly ischaemic heart disease and or heart failure.
- *Ventricular fibrillation* usually results in syncope and sudden death, unless the patient is defibrillated rapidly.
- Untreated, the recurrence rate of VT is high, especially in the presence of impaired systolic function.
- *Symptoms* include palpitations, chest pain, syncope, and presyncope. Sudden cardiac death may be the first symptom.

Causes

In the elderly, VT almost always occurs in the setting of impaired left ventricular function and or ischaemic heart disease. It may be precipitated by electrolyte abnormalities, ischaemia, drugs containing ephedrine or other β-agonists. VT with a normal heart is very rare in the elderly.

Diagnosis

The ECG shows a broad complex tachycardia (Fig. 6.7). Features that help to distinguish VT from SVT with aberrant conduction or BBB are listed in Box 6.4. In patients with intermittent symptoms ambulatory monitoring is required for diagnosis. Repeated monitoring may be required, or in some cases one may consider an implantable loop recorder (see Chapter 8). Elderly patients do not tolerate VT well and therefore symptoms usually correlate with the presence of the arrhythmia.

> **Box 6.4 Differentiating SVT from VT**
>
> Features that favour VT are:
> - QRS of >140 ms
> - Cannon a waves on jugular venous pressure (JVP)
> - Fusion and/or capture beats
> - Dissociated p waves
> - History of ischaemic heart disease
> - Right bundle branch block with left axis deviation
> - Concordance of the QRS complexes in the chest leads
> - Heart rate >170 bpm.

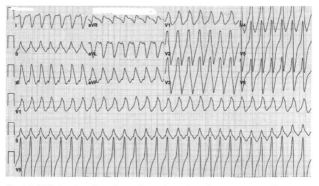

Fig. 6.7 ECG showing a broad complex tachycardia with positive concordance in a 75-year-old man with previous myocardial infarction and impaired left ventricular function. He presented with presyncope and was referred for implantable cardioverter-defibrillator (ICD) implantation. He was treated with β-blockers and had no recurrence of symptoms.

Management

Management options depend on the underlying cause and need to be tailored to the individual. They include:

- Immediate DC cardioversion if the patient is haemodynamically compromised
- Treatment of ischaemia (see Chapter 3)
- Correction of electrolyte imbalance (K^+ and Mg^{2+})
- Optimized treatment for heart failure (see Chapter 5)
- Antiarrhythmic drugs – β-blockers are usually first line. Amiodarone is used if they are contraindicated
- **ICDs**. These are devices which detect abnormal ventricular rates and terminate the arrhythmia according to programmed algorithms. The ICD can terminate abnormal, fast ventricular rates by acting as an 'overdrive' pacemaker, which is known as 'anti-tachycardia pacing'. If repeated bursts of overdrive pacing fail to cardiovert VT, then an electrical shock will be administered. If ventricular fibrillation is detected, electrical defibrillation therapy is delivered. The ICD also has pacemaker capability to deal with slow heart rates. There are NICE guidelines for the use of ICDs (2006) and while some indications are not applicable to elderly patients, they should be considered in those with a reasonable quality of life and prognosis (see Chapter 5 for summary of NICE guidelines).

Torsades de pointes is a type of polymorphic ventricular tachycardia, characterised by beat-to-beat variability of the amplitude and polarity of the QRS complexes.

- It is usually associated with acquired prolongation of the QT interval, >450 msec (Table 6.3).
- Treatment involves elimination of the underlying cause.
- In the acute phase recurrences can be prevented by temporary pacing or isoprenaline infusion.

Table 6.3 Causes of QT prolongation

Electrolyte abnormalities:
Hypokalaemia
Hypocalcaemia
Hypomagnesaemia
Drug induced:
Tricyclic antidepressants (e.g. amitriptyline)
Quinidine
Erythromycin
Antiarrythmics (e.g. amiodarone and sotalol)
Phenothiazines (chlorpropamide)
Antihistamines (terfenadine)
Other causes:
Hypothermia
Hypothyroidism
Grapefruit juice

Indications for referral to an arrhythmia specialist

With improvements in electrophysiology techniques it is likely that more elderly patients will be suitable for device therapy and ablation therapy in the future with lower risk of procedural complications and higher success rates.

At present the following should be referral for specialist advice:
- Palpitation with severe symptoms – syncope or dyspnoea
- Wide QRS complex tachycardia of unknown aetiology especially if poorly tolerated
- Drug resistant or intolerant narrow complex tachycardia
- Tachycardiomyopathy
- WPW – rarely presents *de novo* in elderly.

Important points to remember

- Arrhythmias are a common cause of morbidity and mortality in the elderly.
- They are usually associated with underlying cardiovascular disease.
- Sinus node dysfunction and AV block are common causes of symptomatic bradycardia requiring permanent pacing in the elderly.
- Immediate DC cardioversion is essential in patients with narrow or wide complex tachycardias and haemodynamic compromise.
- Tachyarrhythmias may present with syncope and presyncope rather than palpitation.
- Non-specific symptoms such as weakness and fatigue may occur.
- VT is a complex and serious cardiac arrhythmia in the elderly which should be investigated and managed initially in secondary care setting and referral to an arrhythmia specialist should be considered if ICD implantation is appropriate (see NICE guidelines in Chapter 5).

Guidelines, references, and recommended reading

Gregoratos G, Abrams J, Epstein AE, Freedman RA, Hayes DL, Hlatky MA, *et al.*; American College of Cardiology/American Heart Association Task Force on Practice Guidelines/North American Society for Pacing and Electrophysiology Committee to Update the 1998 Pacemaker Guidelines (2002) ACC/AHA/NASPE 2002 guideline update for implantation of cardiac pacemakers and antiarrhythmia devices: summary article: a report of the American College of Cardiology/American Heart Association Task Force on Practice Guidelines (ACC/AHA/NASPE Committee to Update the 1998 Pacemaker Guidelines). *J Am Coll Cardiol* **106**:(16):2145–61.

National Institute for Health and Clinical Excellence (2005) Dual-chamber pacemakers for symptomatic bradycardia due to sick sinus syndrome and/or atrioventricular block. Technical appraisal guidance 88. London: National Institute for Health and Clinical Excellence. Available from: www.nice.org.uk/TA088

National Institute for Health and Clinical Excellence (2006) Implantable cardioverter defibrillators for arrhythmias. Technology appraisal guidance 95. London: National Institute for Health and Clinical Excellence. Available from: www.nice.org.uk/TA095.

Vaedas PE, Auricchio A, Blanc JJ, Daubert JC, Drexler H, Ector H *et al.* The Task Force for Cardiac Pacing and Resynchronization Therapy of the European Society of Cardiology. Developed in association with the European Heart Rhythm Association (2007). Guidelines for cardiac pacing and cardiac resynchronisation therapy *Eur Heart J* **28**:2256–95.

Atrial fibrillation in the elderly

Epidemiology

- Atrial fibrillation (AF) is the most frequently encountered arrhythmia in the elderly and is usually associated with underlying heart disease.
- The prevalence increases with age, affecting about 10% of those over 80; 70% of patients with AF are over 65 years of age.
- AF is associated with a doubling of cardiovascular mortality.
- Risk of thrombo-embolic stroke is increased up to sevenfold in non-rheumatic AF and 17-fold in rheumatic AF. Annual risk of stroke attributable to AF increases from 1.5% in 50–59 year olds to 23.5% in 80–90 year olds.
- 1 in every 6 strokes occurs in patients with AF, and outcome and mortality are worse than in patients with stroke and sinus rhythm (SR).

Definition

- AF is an irregular, uncoordinated, and rapid beating of the atria resulting in little or no effective mechanical contraction.
- Manifests on electrocardiogram (ECG) as absence of P waves, which are replaced by rapid and irregular oscillations or fibrillatory waves (Fig. 7.1), and an irregular ventricular rhythm, which in the absence of treatment or conduction disease, is usually rapid.

Consequences

The loss of atrial contraction leads to:

- Reduction in cardiac output, which can precipitate or exacerbate heart failure. AF is less well tolerated in the elderly as loss of atrial contraction is more likely to reduce cardiac output when left ventricular filling is impaired e.g. in hypertension, left ventricular hypertrophy, impaired relaxation, and mitral stenosis.
- Atrial thrombus formation that can lead to systemic embolization hence thromboembolic prophylaxis is essential even when SR is restored.
- AF may coexist with conduction system disease or be the first manifestation of sick sinus syndrome (see Bradycardia and AF, p. 163) in the elderly so symptomatic bradycardia is more common.

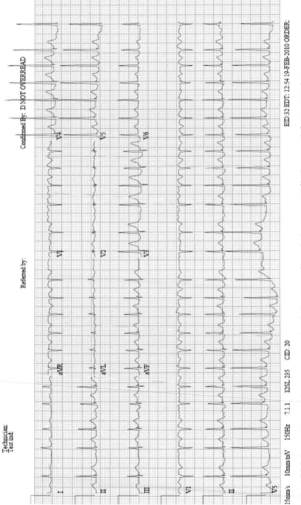

Fig. 7.1 12-lead ECG from a 76-year-olc man presenting with shortness of breath showing atrial fibrilation with fast ventricular rate.

Classification

Initial event: First detected episode. May not be symptomatic and may or may not recur.

Paroxysmal: Terminates spontaneously but recurs. Lasts <7 days and usually less than 48 hours. May progress to persistent or permanent AF.

Persistent: Does not terminate spontaneously. Lasts more than 7 days usually, and requires chemical or electrical cardioversion to restore SR.

Permanent: Longstanding AF, usually >1 year, that fails to cardiovert, relapses after cardioversion, or where cardioversion is felt to be inappropriate. May revert to SR after a disease process is treated (e.g. thyrotoxicosis) or after a specialist procedure to modify the electrophysiological properties of the heart.

Lone: AF occurring without structural heart disease. This is rare in the elderly.

Pathophysiology

AF results from both substrate and a trigger.
- The substrate is most often a pathology affecting the atria, such as hypertensive heart disease (Table 7.1).
- The trigger is usually an ectopic atrial electrical focus, which can arise anywhere in the atria or within the pulmonary vein orifices.
- Once initiated, the arrhythmia is maintained by re-entry circuits that sustain themselves more readily in diseased or enlarged atria.
- The prospect of spontaneous return to SR diminishes with time due to a process of electrical remodelling within the atria.

Table 7.1 Causes of atrial fibrillation

Cardiac	Non-cardiac
Valvular heart disease, especially mitral valve disease	Hyperthyroidism
Ischaemic heart disease including acute coronary syndromes	Alcohol abuse
Hypertension	Infection (especially pneumonia)
Sick sinus syndrome	Pulmonary embolism
Obesity	Bronchial carcinoma
Cardiomyopathy	Electrolyte disturbances
Pericardial disease	Post-thoracotomy
Atrial myxoma	Postoperative
Atrial septal defect	Obesity

Clinical features

History

- Some patients are completely asymptomatic.
- Common symptoms are palpitations, shortness of breath, and fatigue.
- More sinister symptoms are chest pain, dizziness, and syncope, and suggest significant haemodynamic compromise. Syncope may be related to rapid ventricular rates or bradyarrhythmias such as sinus node dysfunction unmasked by treatment.
- Heart failure, cardiac ischaemia, and thrombo-embolic events may be precipitated by AF.

Examination

- Irregularly irregular pulse.
- Record apical rate.
- Auscultate for heart murmurs.
- Look for signs of compromise, e.g. heart failure.

Search for an underlying cause and treat, e.g. ischaemia, valvular heart disease, thyrotoxicosis, lung disease, infection, etc. AF may resolve once the precipitating cause has been treated. Table 7.2 lists the baseline investigations in AF.

Table 7.2 Baseline investigations in atrial fibrillation

Blood tests	FBC, U+E, magnesium, creatinine, TFTs
ECG	Ambulatory ECG may be needed in those with paroxysmal symptoms
CXR	Signs of lung disease e.g. pneumonia
	Evidence of heart failure
Echocardiography/ Doppler	Structural heart disease, e.g. valvular disease, enlarged left atrium, left ventricular function (best performed when the patient has been rate controlled as otherwise difficult to assess ventricular function accurately)
Holter monitoring	This is not essential but may be useful to assess rate control especially if the patient remains symptomatic or if bradyarrhythmias are suspected

CXR, chest radiograph; FBC, full blood count; U+E, urea and electrolytes; TFT, thyroid function test.

Management of the patient with AF

There are three objectives to the management of the patient with AF which are not mutually exclusive:
- Rate control
- Rhythm control
- Prevention of thrombo-embolism.

Factors to consider are:
- Type and duration of AF
- Severity and type of symptoms
- Associated cardiovascular disease and prognosis
- Associated medical conditions and reversible cause (e.g. sepsis, thyrotoxicosis)
- Stroke risk stratification.

The rhythm versus rate control debate and the older patient

Until recently it was assumed that restoring and maintaining SR (rhythm control) was the best management for AF. Five prospective randomized trials have compared the efficacy and safety of rhythm control to rate-control strategies in AF. AFFIRM was the largest of these trials, published in 2002 and is reviewed in Chapter 11 (Wyse *et al.* 2002). Most subjects enrolled in these trials were elderly. All of the studies have failed to show an advantage of one treatment strategy over the other. There are many explanations for this but at present the appropriate strategy in most elderly patients with AF for a number of reasons is rate control (Box 7.1). An attempt at rhythm control may be warranted in patients who are highly symptomatic and where the chances of success are relatively higher: brief history, structurally normal heart, or an acute precipitant. As more effective and less toxic drugs become available for rhythm control, this may be a more feasible option in the elderly.

Box 7.1 Factors favouring a rate-control strategy in the elderly with AF

- AF in the elderly is often due to structural heart disease and likely to recur despite cardioversion.
- AF is frequently established (i.e. permanent) at diagnosis and cardioversion is unlikely to be successful.
- The elderly patient may not tolerate electrical cardioversion due to other co-morbidities.
- AF is non-infrequently associated with acute illness, e.g. sepsis, pneumonia, exacerbation of chronic obstructive pulmonary disease; once acute illness is successfully treated, AF may resolve.
- Even if rhythm control is achieved the current evidence suggests that the risk of thrombo-embolism remains high in many elderly patients so anticoagulation needs to be continued.

Rate control for AF in the elderly

Pharmacological agents are still the mainstay of treatment with β-blockers as first choice agents as outlined in Table 7.3. The role of cardioversion, ablation and pacing in the elderly are discussed on pp.160–2.

Table 7.3 Initial management of atrial fibrillation

Clinical scenario	Treatment
Acute AF and haemodynamically stable	Control rate with a short-acting B-blocker such as intravenous esmolol or oral metoprolol, provided the patient does not have severe heart failure or hypotension (BP <90mmHg systolic). Once the patient has been stabilized switch to once-daily atenolol or bisoprolol
	Rate slowing Ca^{2+} antagonists, verapamil or diltiazem, can be used when B-blockers are contraindicated due to asthma or intolerance, but are also contraindicated in severe heart failure or hypotension
	Digoxin is not negatively inotropic so can be used in heart failure and is less effective but the response is delayed until adequate loading has been achieved
	Treat underlying sepsis/thyrotoxicosis/heart failure and electrolyte and metabolic disturbance
If haemodynamically compromised (systolic BP <90 mmHg that is new for patient, ongoing chest pain, signs of heart failure and impaired conscious level)	Electrical cardioversion (see p. 160) is preferred. Chemical cardioversion with intravenous amiodarone if anaesthesia contraindicated or there is a delay in organizing. Remember amiodarone may lower blood pressure further so careful monitoring and resuscitation are essential. Both options require thrombo-embolic prophylaxis (see Thrombo-embolic prophylaxis, p. 164)
Paroxysmal AF	Cardio-selective β-blocker such as atenolol or bisoprolol as first line
	Sotalol if cardio-selective β-blocker ineffective
	Amiodarone if β-blocker and sotalol ineffective or contraindicated

(Contd.)

Table 7.3 (*Contd.*)

Clinical scenario	Treatment
Persistent AF	Rate-control strategy
	Cardioselective β-blocker as for paroxysmal AF
	Rate slowing Ca^{2+} antagonists such as diltiazem or verapamil can be used as an alternative in asthmatic patients or those who do not tolerate β-blockers due to side effects
	Digoxin is not negatively inotropic so can be used in heart failure and hypotension. However, it is less effective than other agents at controlling exercise induced increases in heart rate. There are also concerns of increased mortality in heart failure. It is only recommended as a sole agent in the sedentary elderly
	If a single agent does not achieve rate control then digoxin may be added to either a β-blocker or Ca^{2+} antagonists but care must be taken in the elderly to avoid inducing symptomatic bradycardia (see p. 163)
	Rhythm control strategy (see p. 160)
	Amiodarone is the most effective agent available in the UK for this. Flecainide and propafenone are contraindicated in the elderly as most elderly patients with AF have underlying heart disease
Permanent AF	Management is the same as for persistent AF

AF, atrial fibrillation; BP, blood pressure.

Drugs used to treat AF in the elderly

- *Amiodarone* may be used to chemically convert AF to SR or to maintain SR in paroxysmal AF (PAF) or after cardioversion. It should not be used for rate control unless all other drugs have failed. It interacts with many drugs (Box 7.2) and has many potential side effects including deranged thyroid function, deranged liver function, pulmonary fibrosis and peripheral neuropathy, and skin and eye problems. Thyroid and liver function tests (TFTs and LFTs) must be checked prior to starting treatment and monitored at 6-monthly intervals thereafter. Amiodarone can prolong the QT interval and cause life-threatening ventricular arrhythmias and can also cause bradycardia. When administered intravenously, care should be taken to minimize risk of extravasation, i.e. give via at least 18 G cannula or preferably a long line (femoral/jugular/subclavian). Intravenous amiodarone acts relatively rapidly but given orally it takes weeks to achieve steady-state levels. The usual intravenous loading dose is 300 mg over 15–30 minutes followed by 900 mg over 24 hours. Oral loading regimens (up to 10 g required) vary but usually take 2–3 weeks (e.g. 200 mg tds for 1 week, 200 mg bd for 1 week and then 200 mg daily). The maintenance dose should be the lowest possible to control the arrhythmia and is usually 100–200 mg daily but 400 mg daily may be required in some patients.

- *β-blockers* are the first-line treatment for AF in most circumstances. In acute AF it is best to start with a short-acting agent such as metoprolol 12.5–25 mg tds and uptitrate according to response. Aim for resting heart rate 60–80, and 90–115 on exertion, depending on symptoms. Once stabilized switch to a once-daily β-blocker, such as atenolol 50–100 mg daily or bisoprolol 2.5–10 mg daily.

- *Sotalol* can be used as an alternative to amiodarone if a standard β-blocker fails to control PAF or to maintain SR after cardioversion. Start with 40 mg twice daily uptitrating to 120 mg twice daily according to response. It can prolong the QT interval and cause life-threatening ventricular arrhythmias.

- *Rate-slowing Ca^{2+} antagonists* are used to control rate if β-blockers are contraindicated and left ventricular systolic function is preserved. Start with diltiazem 60 mg bd or verapamil 40 mg tds and uptitrate according to response. Once-daily slow-release preparations will aid compliance once optimum dose is achieved. Diltiazem is preferred in the elderly by most physicians as it seems to have a better side effect profile.

- *Digoxin* should not be used as a first-line agent to control rate in ambulant patients because it is only effective when the patient is resting, i.e. poor rate control on exertion. It does not prevent AF and therefore has no role in the treatment of paroxysmal AF. After loading with 0.75–1.5 mg over 24 hours, the usual maintenance dose in the elderly is 0.125 mg daily, adjusted according to response and renal function. There is little place for routine measurement of serum levels unless toxicity is suspected (nausea, arrhythmias (e.g. bradycardia), confusion and blurred vision) or there is a lack of response.

Box 7.2 Amiodarone – drug interactions

Amiodarone inhibits the action of the cytochrome P450 isozyme family and reduces the clearance of many drugs, including the following:
- Ciclosporin
- Digoxin
- Flecainide
- Procainamide
- Quinidine
- Sildenafil
- Simvastatin
- Theophylline
- Warfarin.

Rhythm control for AF in the elderly

Cardioversion to achieve rhythm control is required when the patient is haemodynamically compromised and does not respond promptly to pharmacological measures (see Table 7.3). It is also considered electively when:

- Symptoms persist in spite of adequate rate control
- Rate control fails to slow the ventricular rate adequately
- Rate-control agents are not tolerated.

Pharmacological versus electrical cardioversion

- Cardioversion can be achieved by means of drugs or electrical shocks.
- Electrical cardioversion is more likely to be successful but requires sedation or anaesthesia.
- The most effective drug for cardioversion is **amiodarone**, which is associated with significant side effects (see p. 158).
- Other pharmacological agents for cardioversion such as **flecainide** and **propafenone** are contraindicated in patients with underlying heart disease so should be avoided in the elderly.
- **Dronedarone** is a new multichannel-blocking antiarrhythmic drug that has a better side effect profile than amiodarone and reduces cardiovascular morbidity and mortality (see Chapter 11, ATHENA trial) but may be less effective at maintaining SR (DIONYSOS trial – not yet published). The National Institute for Health and Clinical Excellence (NICE) is expected to publish guideline on dronedarone in August 2010. Dronedarone may be considered as an option, within its licensed indications, by specialists for those patients who cannot tolerate amiodarone. Clinicians will need to balance whether dronedarone, a less efficacious but possibly safer antiarrhythmic drug than amiodarone, is justified.
- The risk of thrombo-embolism or stroke is similar for pharmacological and electrical methods of cardioversion so the recommendations for anticoagulation are the same for both methods (see Thrombo-embolic prophylaxis, p. 164).
- A number of initial studies suggest that angiotensin-converting enzyme (ACE) inhibitors and angiotensin II receptor blockers (ARBs) may prevent new onset and recurrent AF. However, the available data do not support the use of these drugs solely for the prevention of AF.

Non-pharmacological management of AF

Electrical cardioversion

- Direct current cardioversion involves delivery of an electrical shock synchronized with the intrinsic activity of the heart by sensing the R wave of the ECG to ensure that electrical stimulation does not occur during the vulnerable period of the cardiac cycle.
- It may be performed acutely in the event of AF resulting in haemodynamic instability or more commonly as an elective procedure with short general anaesthetic in patients who have symptomatic AF (see p. 155, Table 7.3).
- To reduce the number of shocks and myocardial damage, it is recommended to use biphasic waveforms and start with 100 J (max 200 J) especially in chronic AF.
- Current is traditionally delivered through external chest wall electrodes but internal cardiac electrodes are available and may achieve higher success rates in obesity and chronic obstructive pulmonary disease.
- If there is a high risk of cardioversion failure (e.g. previous failed cardioversion), pretreatment with amiodarone may be given. This is usually continued for 3–6 months post procedure if successful, or long term if there is a high risk of relapse (e.g. previous relapse, left atrium (LA) >5 cm, mitral valve disease, >12 months duration of AF, structural heart disease). The benefits of long-term amiodarone therapy need to be balance against the risk of adverse effects in each patient.
- The main complication is thrombo-embolism, so patients require full anticoagulation with warfarin therapy for at least 4 weeks prior to the procedure. In the acute setting, anticoagulation with heparin is recommended although there is little evidence base for this. Anticoagulation should also be continued for 4 weeks post procedure in all patients and then reviewed as many patients will still be at moderate to high risk of thromboembolism and need to continue treatment in the long term.

Radiofrequency ablation

This involves targeted cautery of cardiac tissue by local application of radiofrequency energy. Target zones are identified during an electrophysiological study, in which a series of catheters are placed in the heart. Better understanding of the mechanisms causing AF has stimulated the development of new ablation techniques that target both substrate and trigger. Initial results are promising, but long-term data and studies in diseased hearts and the elderly are needed. It is not first line treatment and at present it is only recommended for (NICE 2006a):

- Patients with paroxysmal AF if antiarrhythmic drugs are ineffective or not tolerated

- Highly selected patients with permanent or persistent AF who are refractory to and or intolerant of medical treatment (refer for specialist advice).

Ablation and cardiac pacing

- Atrioventricular junction (AVJ) catheter ablation and pacing is another treatment option. This is based on the principle that a regular ventricular rhythm will improve symptoms and haemodynamic performance
- Studies to date are small and not specific to the elderly. Meta-analysis suggests improvement in symptoms, exercise tolerance, cardiac physiology and function, and reduced hospital admissions.
- At present it is only recommended for patients with drug-resistant, poorly tolerated AF.

Surgery for AF

The modified Maze procedure involves creating atrial incisions at critical locations to create barriers to conduction and prevent sustained AF. Radiofrequency ablation is now used as an alternative to surgical incisions. Cardiopulmonary bypass is required so it is rarely undertaken as a primary procedure in the UK, but it should be considered if the patient is having cardiac surgery for valve disease or ischaemic heart disease. High success rates are reported in patients having mitral valve surgery. Success rates in the elderly are unknown.

Bradycardia and AF

Bradycardia can occur in patients in AF either as a cause of the arrhythmia or as a result of the treatment for the arrhythmia.

- Patients with **sick sinus syndrome/sinus node disease** are more likely to have AF, presumably because the pauses enhance the occurrence of atrial premature beats which initiate the arrhythmia. Some studies suggest a reduction in AF by atrial or physiological pacing.
- Both rate-control drugs and drugs used to maintain SR can cause bradycardia by suppressing the sinus node or by aggravating heart block.
- Regardless of the aetiology, patients who develop symptomatic bradycardia or significant pauses usually require permanent pacing.

Thrombo-embolic prophylaxis

This is a key consideration in the management of AF because AF, whether paroxysmal, persistent or permanent, carries an equal and significant risk of stroke. The commonest used tool for guiding stroke risk stratification in patients with AF is the CHADS2 score.

Table 7.4 CHADS2 score

Factor	Score
Congestive heart failure	1
Hypertension	1
Age >75	1
Diabetes	1
Stroke or transient ischaemic attack in past	2

Annual stroke risk is doubled with a score of 2 and increases further with higher scores. Patients with a score of 1 or 2 should therefore be treated with warfarin or aspirin. Those with a score of 3 or more should be anticoagulated with warfarin unless the risks significantly outweigh the benefits.

One of the difficulties is that elderly patients who are at greatest risk of bleeding with anticoagulation are those who get the most benefit. Haemorrhagic prediction scores have been developed to help predict risk of bleeding (Table 7.5).

Table 7.5 HEMORR2HAGES score to predict risk of major bleeding on warfarin for atrial fibrillation

Score	Major bleeding per 100 person-years (95% CI)
0	1.9 (0.6–4.4)
1	2.5 (1.3–4.3)
2	5.3 (3.4–8.1)
3	8.4 (4.9–13.6)
4	10.4 (5.1–18.9)
≥5	12.3 (5.8–23.1)

The HEMORR2HAGES score is calculated by adding 1 point for each of the following: hepatic or renal disease, ethanol abuse, malignancy, age >75 years, reduced platelet count or function, uncontrolled hypertension, anaemia, excess falls risk, and stroke, and 2 points for prior bleed (Gage et al. 2006).

Contraindications to warfarin therapy

- History of intracerebral haemorrhage
- Recent peptic ulceration (in last 12 months. Need endoscopic evidence of healing prior to anticoagulation with either aspirin or warfarin)
- Recent stroke (<2 weeks).

Cautions in warfarin therapy

These include:

- Recurrent falls
- Cognitive impairment
- Unexplained anaemia
- Concurrent use of non-steroidal anti-inflammatory drugs (NSAIDs), aspirin or other antiplatelet agents
- Uncontrolled hypertension
- Patients on multiple medications – increased risk of drug interactions and adverse events.

The decision on anticoagulation needs to be made for each individual patient taking the above factors into consideration. The target INR is 2.5 with range 2–3.

Despite the higher risk associated with stroke in the elderly, thromboprophylaxis for AF is suboptimal. This is partly because of the perceived increased risk associated with co-morbidity, interactions with concomitant drug therapies and bleeding, and also patient factors whereby some patients decline the most effective treatment option.

The BAFTA study (see Chapter 11) shows that warfarin is 65% more effective than aspirin in reducing risk of stroke in elderly patients with AF with no significant difference in bleeding risk.

The elderly are more sensitive to warfarin than younger patients. Factors influencing the pharmacokinetics of warfarin are not age-specific and are listed in Table 7.6. The pharmacodynamic response to warfarin is increased in the elderly for the reasons listed in Table 7.6. Lower loading and maintenance doses are therefore recommended in the elderly (refer to local guidelines).

Table 7.6 Factors affecting the pharmacokinetics and pharmacodynamics of warfarin in the elderly

Pharmacokinetics	Pharmacodynamics
Decreased absorption (fat malabsorption, cholestyramine)	Decreased synthesis of clotting factors due to liver disease
Genetic enzyme polymorphisms affecting hepatic metabolism	Low dietary vitamin K intake (leafy green vegetables)
Drug interactions at the CYP2C9 level that can increase or decrease INR level	Level of vitamin K produced by intestinal bacteria may be decreased by broad spectrum antibiotics
Frequent changes to concomitant medication due to intercurrent illness	Concomitant use of drugs interfering with platelet function (aspirin, clopidogrel, NSAIDs)
	Hypermetabolic states such as fever may increase response to warfarin (possibly due to increased catabolism of Vitamin K dependent factors)

INR, international normalized ratio; NSAID, non-steroidal anti-inflammatory drug.

Alternatives to warfarin and the future

There is little evidence regarding aspirin dosage in the treatment of AF. The NICE guidelines recommend 75–300 mg daily. Considerations regarding dosage should include a history of peptic ulceration and bleeding risk and if this is significant lower doses are recommended.

At present there is no evidence that the combination of aspirin and fixed dose warfarin, clopidogrel alone or in combination with aspirin, or dipyridamole are superior to adjusted dose warfarin in patients with AF.

New antithrombotic agents are currently available but not yet in widespread clinical use and guidance on their role in AF is awaited. Dabigatran, a new oral direct thrombin inhibitor, appears to be as effective as warfarin in reducing risk of stroke in patients with AF with lower bleeding risk (Re-LY, see Chapter 11). NICE Guidelines are expected in 2011.

Another oral direct thrombin inhibitor, ximelagatran, also appears to be as effective as warfarin for prevention of stroke and systemic embolism in patients with AF with lower bleeding risk but there are concerns regarding hepatotoxicity (SPORTIF V, see Chapter 11). The advantages of these new agents are that they do not require loading or monitoring and drug interactions are less frequent than with warfarin therapy. Hence, they may prove particularly useful in the elderly.

Percutaneous occlusion of the left atrial appendage is a relatively new technique that may be considered an alternative to prevent thrombo-embolic complications in patients with non-valvular AF and contraindications to anticoagulation with warfarin. It is currently being reviewed by NICE (see www.nice.org.uk/IPG181) but studies to date are small and short term.

Important points to remember

- Most patients with AF are over 65 years of age.
- AF is an important cause of morbidity and mortality in the elderly.
- At present there is no evidence that rhythm control is superior to rate control.
- Anticoagulation to reduce thrombo-embolic risk is an essential part of management.

Guidelines, references, and recommended reading

Albers GW, Diener HC, Frison L, Grind M, Nevinson M, Partridge S, et al.; SPORTIF Executive Steering Committee for the SPORTIF V Investigators (2005) Ximelagatran vs warfarin for stroke prevention in patients with nonvalvular atrial fibrillation. A randomized trial. *JAMA* **293**: 690–8.

Connolly SJ, Ezekowitz MD, Yusuf S, Eikelboom J, Oldgren J, Parekh A, et al.; RE-LY Steering Committee and Investigators (2009) Dabigatran versus warfarin in patients with atrial fibrillation (Re-LY). *N Engl J Med* **361**:1139–51.

Fuster V, Rydén LE, Cannom DS, Crijns HJ, Curtis AB, Ellenbogen KA, et al.; American College of Cardiology; American Heart Association Task Force; European Society of Cardiology Committee for Practice Guidelines; European Heart Rhythm Association; Heart Rhythm Society (2006) ACC/AHA/ESC 2006 guidelines for the management of patients with atrial fibrillation: full text: a report of the American College of Cardiology/American Heart Association Task Force on practice guidelines and the European Society of Cardiology Committee for Practice Guidelines (Writing Committee to Revise the 2001 guidelines for the management of patients with atrial fibrillation) developed in collaboration with the European Heart Rhythm Association and the Heart Rhythm Society. *Europace* **8**:651–745.

Gage BF, Yan Y, Milligan PE, Waterman AD, Culverhouse R, Rich MW, Radford MJ (2006) Clinical classification schemes for predicting hemorrhage: results from the National Registry of Atrial Fibrillation (NRAF). *Am Heart J* **151**:713–19.

Hohnloser SH, Crijns HJ, van Eickels M, Gaudin C, Page RL, Torp-Pedersen C, et al.; ATHENA Investigators (2009) Effect of dronedarone on cardiovascular events in atrial fibrillation. *N Engl J Med* **360**:668–78.

National Institute for Health and Clinical Excellence (2006a) Percutaneous radiofrequency ablation for atrial fibrillation. Interventional procedure guidance 168. London: National Institute for Health and Clinical Excellence. Available from www.nice.org.uk/IPG168.

National Institute for Health and Clinical Excellence (2006b) The management of atrial fibrillation. Clinical guideline 36. London: National Institute for Health and Clinical Excellence. Available from: www.nice.org.uk/CG036.

Wyse DG, Waldo AL, DiMarco JP, Domanski MJ, Rosenberg Y, Schron EB, et al. A comparison of rate control and rhythm control in patients with atrial fibrillation. The Atrial Fibrillation Follow-up Investigation of Rhythm Management (AFFIRM) study. *N Engl J Med* **347**:1825–33.

Chapter 8

Syncope and orthostatic (postural) hypotension

Definitions

Syncope is a sudden, transient loss of consciousness associated with loss of postural tone with spontaneous recovery. It usually results from cerebral hypoperfusion.

Presyncope is a milder disorder without loss of consciousness. It is characterized by transient weakness, light-headedness, reduced awareness of surroundings, and an inability to interact.

Epidemiology

- Syncope is common.
- 3% of accident and emergency attendances and 1–6% of hospital admissions.
- Prevalence increases with age. Annual incidence is 6–7% over the age of 75 years.
- Prognosis depends on the underlying cause. Cardiac causes having the worst prognosis with 1-year mortality up to 30%.
- Recurrence rates of 35% over 3 years.
- The rate of injury per syncopal episode is high in the elderly. Injuries such as fractures or subdural haematomas are associated with significant mortality and morbidity irrespective of the cause of syncope. Loss of confidence, fear of recurrence, and depression lead to increasing dependence and institutionalization.

Causes of syncope

The causes of syncope are listed in Table 8.1. Cardiovascular causes of syncope become increasingly common in those over 65 years of age. The commonest causes of syncope in older adults are orthostatic hypotension (up to 30%), cardioinhibitory carotid sinus hypersensitivity (20%), neurally mediated syncope (15%), and cardiac arrhythmias (20%).

Table 8.1 Causes of syncope in the elderly

Cardiac causes
Organic heart disease (valve disease, ischaemia)
Arrhythmias and conduction system disorders
Neurally mediated
Vasovagal
Situational
Cough
Swallow
Micturition
Defecation
Carotid sinus hypersensitivity
Orthostatic hypotension
Neurological
Epilepsy
Transient ischaemic attacks
Migraine
Subclavian steal
Metabolic and endocrine disorders
Hypoglycaemia
Addison's disease
Electrolyte disorders

Syncope of cardiac origin

There are two principal mechanisms:
- Obstruction of cardiac output due to restricted emptying or filling of the ventricle (obstructive syncope – see Table 8.2). The commonest reason for obstructive syncope in the elderly is aortic stenosis. This is discussed in Chapter 3.
- Reduction in cardiac output due to disturbances in cardiac rhythm (arrhythmic syncope, see Table 8.3). Brady-arrhythmias predominate in the elderly. Arrhythmias are discussed in Chapter 6.
- Less commonly, syncope may occur as a result of an embolus from the heart obstructing cerebral blood flow or from aortic dissection.

Table 8.2 Cardiac disorders associated with obstructive syncope

Aortic stenosis
Hypertrophic cardiomyopathy
Mitral stenosis
Atrial myxoma
Pulmonary hypertension
Pulmonary embolism
Cardiac tamponade
Prosthetic valve malfunction

Table 8.3 Cardiac disorders associated with arrhythmic syncope

Bradyarrhythmia

Sinus node dysfunction

  Sinus bradycardia

  Sinus arrest

  Brady-tachy syndrome

Atrioventricular (AV) conduction defect

  2nd degree AV block (Wenckebach)

  2nd degree AV block (Mobitz II)

Complete heart block

Tachyarrhythmia

Supraventricular tachyarrhythmia

  AV nodal node re-entrant tachycardia

  AV tachycardia with Wolff–Parkinson–White

Atrial tachycardia
Atrial flutter

Atrial fibrillation

Ventricular tachycardia

  Monomorphic ventricular tachycardia

  Polymorphic ventricular tachycardia

  Ventricular fibrillation

Pacemaker malfunction

Bradycardia due to:

    Battery failure

    Generator failure

    Electrode dysfunction

    Interference (myopotential or electromagnetic)

    Inappropriate programming

    Pacemaker-mediated tachycardia

    Pacemaker syndrome

Neurally mediated syncope

This results from reflex mechanisms that are associated with inappropriate vasodilatation, bradycardia, or both and includes vasovagal, situational syncope, and carotid sinus hypersensitivity.

Vasovagal syncope

- Loss of consciousness due to neurally mediated hypotension, sometimes accompanied by bradycardia.
- Found in about 15% of elderly patients with syncope.
- There is an inappropriate or paradoxical increase in vagal tone (Bezold–Jarisch reflex) resulting in hypotension and/or bradycardia.
- Classic vagal prodrome of abdominal discomfort, nausea, diaphoresis, visual disturbance, light-headedness.
- Bystanders observe pallor and ashen complexion.
- Urinary incontinence and tonic–clonic muscular contractions may occur.
- Recovery is usually rapid but patients may complain of fatigue that can last up to 1 day.
- In the elderly atypical symptoms or associated co-morbidity may make the diagnosis more difficult and provocative tests may be necessary.
- Head-up tilt testing is an established method of provoking vasovagal responses (Box 8.2).

Situational syncope

The diagnosis of situational syncope is confirmed by the history in most cases.

- *Micturition syncope* typically occurs in elderly men, often in the setting of nocturia and associated with voiding large volumes of urine or consuming large volumes of alcohol.
- *Cough syncope* is associated with protracted spasms of coughing.
- *Defecation syncope* is often associated with straining at stool.
- *Deglutition syncope* is associated with swallowing.
- *Postprandial syncope* is due to a fall in blood pressure typically occurring 30–90 minutes after a meal. It is often associated with postural hypotension and though to be mediated by vasoactive peptides.

Carotid sinus hypersensitivity (CSH)

- Found in 20% or more of elderly patients with syncope.
- Diagnosed by carotid sinus massage (see Physical examination, p. 178).
- CSH represents an exaggerated response to stimulation of the carotid sinus with resultant bradycardia or hypotension or a combination of both (see carotid sinus massage in Physical examination, p. 178).
- Symptoms are classically associated with actions that result in mechanical stimulation of the carotid sinus such as rapid head turning, especially with a tight collar. However, in the majority of patients no precipitating cause can be identified.
- CSH is an important cause of unexplained falls with or without syncope in the elderly.
- 50% of patients with unexplained falls and CSH have amnesia for loss of consciousness.

Investigation of the patient with syncope

See Figure 8.1.

The aim of investigation is to identify the underlying cause to determine the risk of further events and future management. Precise diagnosis of syncope is especially difficult in the elderly due to frequent co-morbidity, diminished reliability of event recall and atypical presentation. Guidelines for the investigation and management of syncope in adults are available and have been incorporated here with specific recommendations for the elderly. Over a third of older people will have more than one possible attributable cause. If symptoms continue or more than one cause is suspected further evaluation is necessary.

History

It is important to get an accurate history of the episode and a witnessed account if possible. Characteristically, patients give a history of sudden loss of consciousness for a brief period with rapid recovery. In contrast, neurological syncope often leaves a residual deficit or period of confusion or drowsiness lasting minutes or hours. Elderly patients often have poor recall for the event and not infrequently have amnesia for loss of consciousness. The presence of structural heart disease has the highest sensitivity for identifying patients with cardiac syncope, but nearly 50% of older patients with heart disease have neurally mediated syncope. Convulsive syncope where there are short-lived myoclonic jerks is often misdiagnosed as epilepsy. Gait and balance instability are common in the elderly and haemodynamic changes insufficient to cause syncope may result in falls.

Important points to enquire about in the history
- Symptoms preceding and following syncope (palpitation, dizziness, chest pain, drowsiness, any focal neurological deficits, etc.).
- Position (supine, sitting, standing) and time of day.
- Relationship of syncope to activity (exertion, micturition, posture change, cough, meals).
- Predisposing factors.
- Associated symptoms (nausea, vomiting, abdominal discomfort, sweating, aura, blurred vision, pain in neck and shoulders, urinary/faecal incontinence).
- Eyewitness should be asked about way of falling, skin colour (pale, flushed, cyanosed), duration of loss of consciousness, movements during syncope and their duration, recovery pattern.
- Any previous cardiac history or previous episodes of syncope and presyncope.
- Medication use and relationship of syncope to timing of medication (medications frequently cause or contribute to syncope in the elderly).

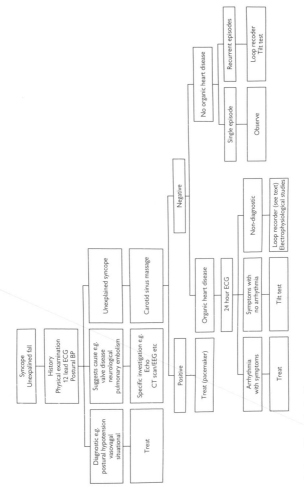

Fig. 8.1 Investigation of the patient with syncope.

Conditions mimicking syncope that are import to exclude are:
- Metabolic disorders (hypoxia, hypocarbia, hypoglycaemia)
- Epilepsy
- Drug intoxication
- Vertebrobasilar insufficiency (will be preceded or accompanied by other brainstem symptoms such as diplopia, dysarthria, etc.)
- Drop attacks (a specific and benign syndrome in which the person, often female, falls to their knees without loss of consciousness)
- Psychogenic (usually witnessed and not associated with injury and rare in the elderly)
- Anxiety/panic disorder.

Syncope – when to admit
- Abnormal electrocardiogram (ECG) (complete heart block, ventricular tachycardia, long QT)
- Previous malignant arrhythmias
- Exertional syncope
- Syncope causing serious injury
- Frequent episodes
- Focal neurological signs.

Physical examination
This is important to detect abnormalities such as aortic stenosis, carotid stenosis, neurological deficits, etc. Arrhythmias such as bradycardias may be detected but are frequently intermittent. Postural blood pressure measurement is important to detect postural hypotension (see below).

12-lead ECG: This may reveal the cause of syncope if the arrhythmia responsible is present at the time of ECG recording. In most cases (>95%) however, this does not happen. Clues as to the cause of syncope may be found, however, such as:
- Sinus bradycardia, AV conduction defects or bifascicular block (Fig. 8.2)
- Pre-excitation of the QRS
- Prolonged QT
- Evidence of previous myocardial infarction or ischaemia.

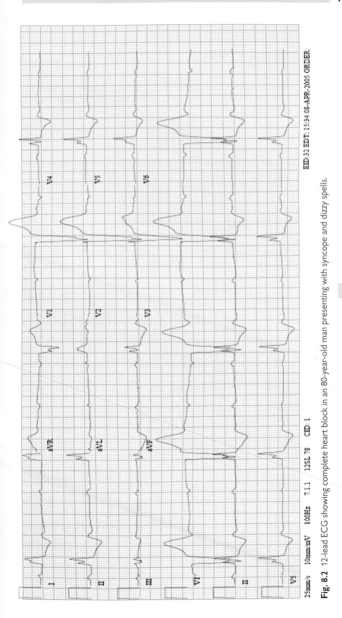

Fig. 8.2 12-lead ECG showing complete heart block in an 80-year-old man presenting with syncope and dizzy spells.

Blood tests are indicated if anaemia, electrolyte disturbances, or hypoglycaemia are likely as indicated by the history and physical examination. The role of biomarkers such as troponin T or I in the diagnostic evaluation of syncope in the emergency department remains unclear and these tests should be performed if clinically indicated (e.g. associated chest pain/dyspnoea/ECG changes of ischaemia). A short Synacthen test is indicated in patients with significant postural hypotension due to autonomic failure.

Carotid sinus massage is a useful initial investigation in elderly patients with syncope or unexplained falls (Box 8.1).

- Carotid sinus hypersensitivity is diagnosed if massage of the carotid sinus produces more than 3 seconds of asystole (cardioinhibitory) (Fig. 8.3) or more than 50 mmHg drop in systolic blood pressure (vasodepressor) either in the supine or head-up tilted position.
- A mixed cardioinhibitory and vasodepressor response can also occur.
- It is contraindicated in patients with carotid disease, recent stroke or myocardial infarction, and ventricular tachycardia.
- About 20% of elderly patients with syncope have a cardioinhibitory response.
- A vasodepressor response is found in another 15–20%, but its role in causing syncope is less clear. However, it does at least warrant a review of medication.

Box 8.1 Protocol for carotid sinus massage

- Lie patient supine for 5 minutes with blood pressure and ECG monitoring on a tilt table.
- Perform firm longitudinal massage for 5 seconds over the site of maximal pulsation of the right carotid sinus (located between the superior border of the thyroid cartilage and the angle of the mandible).
- Record blood pressure (BP) and maximum RR interval. Record any symptoms such as dizziness etc. at each stage. Massage should be discontinued if asystole greater than 3 seconds occurs.
- If right-sided massage is not diagnostic, the procedure should be repeated in the left supine position after haemodynamic equilibration.
- If massage in the supine position is not diagnostic, the procedure should be repeated in the 60° head-up tilt position on the right and left side.
- At the end of the procedure the patient should remain supine for 10 minutes (to reduce risk of neurological complications).
- Stroke and transient ischaemic attack are rare complications. If neurological signs ensue return patient to supine position and take measures to restore BP to normotensive levels. Give aspirin 300 mg unless contraindicated.
- Ventricular and atrial arrhythmias are reported rarely. Resuscitation facilities should be immediately available.

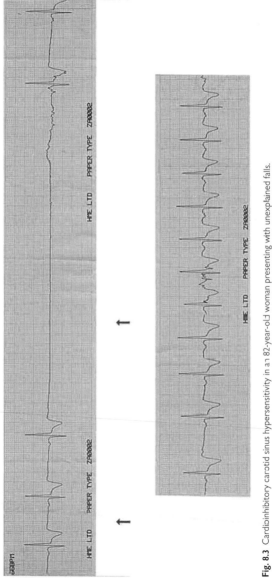

Fig. 8.3 Cardioinhibitory carotid sinus hypersensitivity in an 82-year-old woman presenting with unexplained falls.

A detailed history, clinical examination, ECG, orthostatic blood pressure measurement and supine and upright carotid sinus massage will achieve a diagnosis in about 50% of elderly patients with syncope. If the diagnosis remains elusive, referral for further assessment including ambulatory monitoring, tilt testing, etc. should be considered. Brain imaging, electroencephalograms (EEGs), and carotid Doppler studies are rarely useful unless there are other neurological symptoms and signs.

Ambulatory 24-hour ECG monitoring: This may reveal brady or tachyarrhythmias. However, syncopal episodes are often infrequent and unpredictable and it is often difficult to establish the relationship between an arrhythmia and syncope despite repeated ambulatory ECG recordings. Diagnostic arrhythmias are found in about 4% (Fig. 8.4). Indications for 24-hour monitoring are:

• Symptoms suggestive of arrhythmia (palpitation, sudden loss of consciousness, use of medication associated with arrhythmia)
• Abnormal resting ECG especially conduction abnormalities or arrhythmia
• Known organic heart disease.

Echocardiography and Doppler: This is indicated if aortic stenosis or cardiac embolism is suspected as a cause of syncope.

Exercise testing and cardiac catheterization are unlikely to establish a diagnosis in the evaluation of syncope except exercise testing may be useful when the patient presents with exertional syncope.

Head-up tilt testing: In patients with unexplained syncope, reproduction of symptoms accompanied by tilt induced hypotension and less frequently bradycardia constitute a diagnosis of vasovagal syncope (Box 8.2). However, in the absence of premonitory symptoms it is more difficult to ascertain if the hypotension (Fig. 8.5) and/or bradycardia provoked by tilting are responsible for the syncopal episode.

Box 8.2 Protocol for head-up tilt testing

• Quiet environment with subdued lighting.
• Heart rate and BP monitored continuously.
• Supine resting period for 10 minutes.
• Head-up tilt to 60° for 20 minutes.
• Discontinue if patient becomes syncopal or presyncopal.
• Return to supine position and record BP and pulse until symptoms resolve.
• If negative consider glyceryl trinitrate (GTN) provocation.

External loop or event recorders: These allow monitoring over several days to weeks but require patient activation once a syncopal episode occurs so compliance rates are often poor in the elderly.

Implantable loop recorders: These are devices that are implanted subcutaneously for several months and analyse cardiac rhythm continuously.

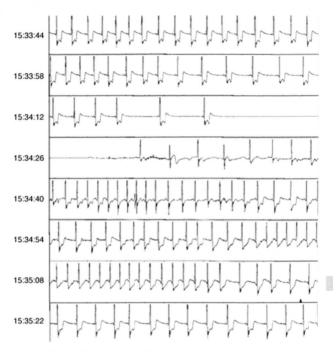

Fig. 8.4 24-hour Holter monitoring showing prolonged sinus pause in a 78-year-old woman presenting with recurrent syncope.

Loop recorders are useful in the patient with recurrent syncope of likely cardiac origin if other investigations prove negative. When activated by the patient or carer they can store cardiac rhythm for subsequent review (Fig. 8.6).

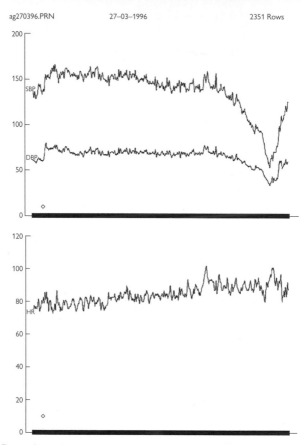

Fig. 8.5 Beat to beat monitoring of heart rate and blood pressure during head-up tilt test performed for investigation of syncope in a 72-year-old woman who presented with recurrent syncopal episodes. As the heart rate increased the patient started to experience her usual prodrome (darkening of vision and feeling the need for air) and lost consciousness briefly as her blood pressure dropped. She recovered rapidly as her blood pressure increased. This confirms vasovagal syncope.

Electrophysiological studies: Patients with a high probability of cardiac syncope who remain undiagnosed after non-invasive testing may require electrophysiological testing to assess sinus node function, AV conduction, and inducibility of ventricular and supraventricular arrhythmias. It is rarely useful in patients with syncope and no underlying heart disease. Even in those with underlying heart disease yields are poor.

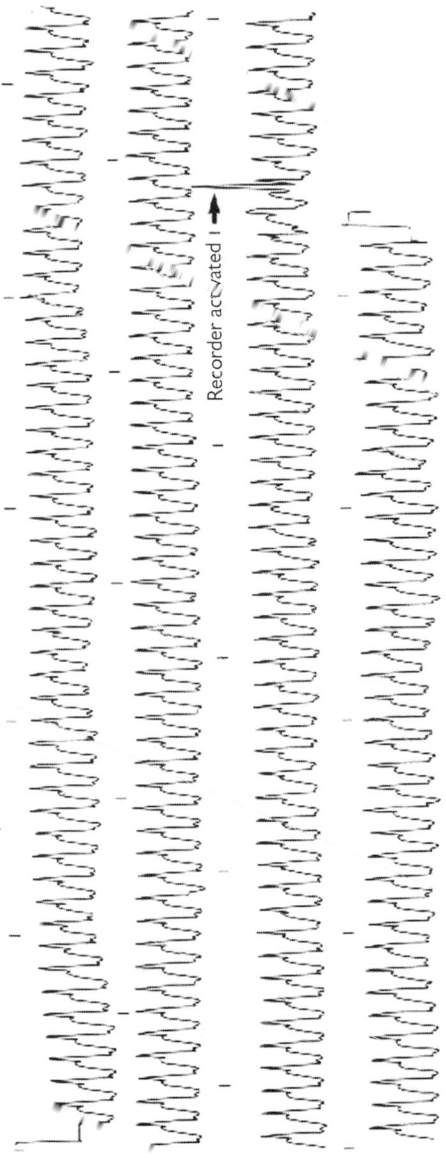

Fig. 8.6 Print out from a Reveal device in a 75-year-old man with recurrent syncope showing ventricular tachycardia recorded during a syncopal episode.

Management of the patient with syncope

- Management depends on the underlying cause.
- The management of valvular heart disease and tachycardias are outlined in Chapters 3 and 6.
- Permanent pacing is indicated for patients with bradycardia-induced syncope and cardioinhibitory CSH and is also beneficial in elderly patients with unexplained falls and cardioinhibitory CSH.
- Management of vasovagal syncope is complex and requires specialist supervision. Non-pharmacological measures include avoiding triggers, recognizing the warning prodrome, reviewing medication, and support stockings are all important. β-Blockers, sympathomimetic agents (ephedrine or midodrine), serotonin selective reuptake inhibitors (SSRIs), and fludrocortisone have varying success rates in individual patients. Permanent pacing may be indicated in some patients if the drop in blood pressure is accompanied by a significant bradycardia.
- The management of postural hypotension is discussed below.
- Patients with syncope should not drive until the cause has been identified and treated (see the Driver and Vehicle Licensing Agency (DVLA) regulations, available from: www.dft.gov.uk).

Evaluation of the frail elderly

Age *per se* is not a contraindication to assessment and intervention but in very frail patients prognosis and compliance with tests as well as the potential benefit to the patient must be considered. Orthostatic blood pressure measurement and carotid sinus massage are usually well tolerated even in frailer patients so can be performed if clinically indicated. There is some evidence that modification of cardiovascular risk factors for falls and syncope reduces the incidence of subsequent events in community dwelling frail patients even with dementia, but to date there is little evidence of benefit in the institutionalized elderly. There is no evidence to date that treatment of hypotension or arrhythmias affects cognitive decline in patients with dementia.

Important points to remember

- Syncope is common in the elderly and may result in serious injury.
- Amnesia for loss of consciousness is common in the elderly.
- Cardiovascular causes of syncope become increasingly common with age.
- Careful history, physical examination, and ECG are important tools in diagnosis.
- Neurological testing is rarely helpful in the absence of additional neurological symptoms and signs.
- Syncope in the elderly may result from medication and abnormal physiological responses to daily events.

Orthostatic (postural) hypotension

- Orthostatic (postural) hypotension is defined as drop of 20 mmHg or more in standing systolic blood pressure or 10 mmHg or more in standing diastolic blood pressure.
- Prevalence increases with age and is reported to be between 5% and 30% in the elderly. This wide variation reflects differences in evaluation methods, definitions, and populations studied.
- It is associated with an increased risk of falls and fractures.
- On standing there is rapid displacement of about 10% of the blood volume from the thorax to the lower body. The normal physiological response to maintain blood pressure involves the neuroendocrine system, baroreflex function, and B-adrenergic responses. With increasing age these responses are decreased, resulting in a fall in blood pressure on standing.
- Progressive orthostatic hypotension is characterized by a slow progressive decrease in systolic blood pressure with a compensatory increase in heart rate on assuming the upright posture. Symptoms tend to occur after a few minutes of standing rather than immediately. It is mainly seen in the elderly and is associated with other co-morbidities and use of vasoactive drugs. It can be diagnosed by tilt testing (see Box 8.2).

Symptoms

Patients may be asymptomatic. Usual symptoms upon standing include:
- Dizziness
- Visual disturbances
- Presyncope or syncope
- Unexplained falls
- Loss of balance and/or unsteadiness
- Neck pain.

Diagnosis

The diagnosis can be confirmed by measuring blood pressure after 5 minutes of lying supine, followed by measurements each minute or more often after standing for 3–5 minutes. If the blood pressure is still falling at 3 minutes monitoring should be continued for longer. If the patient cannot tolerate standing for this period the lowest upright pressure should be recorded or the measurements can be performed using a tilt table. The postural changes are usually most marked in the morning. In patients with autonomic failure, the circadian changes in blood pressure are the reverse of normal and may be detected by 24-hour ambulatory monitoring; supine blood pressure is lowest in the morning and rises gradually during the day. Other important features of autonomic failure are postprandial hypotension and exercise-induced hypotension.

Causes

Medication is the commonest contributing factor to orthostatic hypotension in the elderly. The drugs are listed in Table 8.4. Other neurogenic and non-neurogenic causes are listed in Table 8.5.

Table 8.4 Medication associated with orthostatic (postural) hypotension

Anti-hypertensive drugs
β-blockers
α-blockers
Angiotensin-converting enzyme inhibitors
Angiotensin II receptor blockers
Calcium channel blockers
Vasodilator antihypertensives
Diuretics
Loop diuretics
Thiazides
Potassium-sparing diuretics
Vasodilators
Nitrates
Potassium channel activators
Antidepressants
Tricyclic antidepressants
Selective serotonin reuptake inhibitors
Serotonin and noradrenaline reuptake inhibitors
Antiparkinsonian medication
Levodopa and dopamine receptor antagonists

Table 8.5 Causes of orthostatic (postural) hypotension

Drugs (see Table 8.4)
Neurogenic
Primary
Pure autonomic failure
Shy–Drager Syndrome (combination of multisystem atrophy with autonomic failure)
Autonomic failure and Parkinson's disease
Secondary
Spinal cord lesions (syringobulbia, syringomyelia, cord transection, transverse myelitis, amyloid)
Diabetes mellitus
Old age
Non-neurogenic
Low intravascular volume (fluid loss, renal or endocrine disorders)
Vasodilation (hyperpyrexia, alcohol)

Management
- Review medication.
- Correct hypovolaemia, dehydration, and hyponatraemia if present.
- Non-pharmacological measures that may be helpful in some patients are listed in Table 8.6.
- Medication – there is no specific treatment.
  - Low dose mineralocorticoids such as fludrocortisone 0.1 mg may be beneficial and work by increasing plasma volume and sensitizing the α-receptors. Fluid retention and hypertension are limiting factors.
  - Midodrine, an α-agonist has shown promising results in small studies but its use is limited by systemic vasoconstriction and hypertension. It is only available on a named patient basis in the UK. Start with low doses (2.5 mg tds) and uptitrate according to response to maximum 10 mg qds – last dose should be before 6 pm and it is important to check for supine hypertension. Midodrine is not recommended in patients with systolic BP ≥160 mmHg.
  - Desmopressin (1-desamino-8-D-arginine vasopressin (DDAVP)) may be useful in patients with autonomic failure but hyponatraemia may limit its use.
  - Remember in most cases treatment increases both the resting and standing blood pressure but does not eliminate the postural drop. Increasing the standing blood pressure often eliminates symptoms.

Table 8.6 Non-pharmacological measures for orthostatic (postural) hypotension

Full length elastic stockings
Abdominal binders
Increases caffeine intake
Increased salt and water consumption
Exercise programmes (focusing on balance and gait)
Head-up tilt at night
Small frequent meals Ice cold water ingestion
Avoid
Sudden head-up posture change
Prolonged recumbency
Straining during micturition or defecation
High temperature environments (incl hot baths)
Alcohol
Vasodepressor drugs

Important points to remember

- Orthostatic (postural) hypotension is common in the elderly and is associated with syncope, presyncope, and an increased risk of falls.
- Medication is the commonest contributing factor.
- Medication review is the most important aspect of management.
- Non-pharmacological measures are important to reduce the risk of syncope and falls.

Guidelines

European Society of Cardiology guidelines on management of syncope. Update 2009. European Heart Journal, 2009, **30**:2631–2671. www.escardio.org/guidelines

American Heart Association/American College of Cardiology Foundation Scientific statement on the evaluation of syncope. *J Am Coll Cardiol*, 2006, **47**:473–484. www.americanheart.org

Drivers Medical Group (2010) At a glance guide to the current medical standards of fitness to drive. Swansea: DVLA. Available from: www.dft.gov.uk.

Kenny R, O'Shea D, Parry S (2000) The Newcastle protocols for head-up tilt table testing in the diagnosis of vasovagal syncope, carotid sinus hypersensitivity, and related disorders. *Heart* **83**: 564–569.

Romero-Ortuno R and Kenny RA. (2008) Is it cardiac? Assessment of syncope with a scoring system. *Heart*, **94**:1528–1529.

Chapter 9

Hypertension in the elderly

Definition

Blood pressure has a unimodal distribution in the population and the relationship between cardiovascular risk and blood pressure is continuous, so there is no critical level above which the risk suddenly increases. Nonetheless in order to facilitate management, current guidelines use arbitrary cut-off values for classification of systolic-diastolic hypertension (Table 9.1).

Epidemiology

- The prevalence of hypertension increases with age—at least 60% of those >65 years or older have hypertension or are receiving antihypertensive treatment.
- The lifetime risk of developing hypertension among 55–65-year-old individuals in the Framingham Heart Study is >90%.
- In 2002 the World Health Organization (WHO) listed hypertension as the most important preventable cause of death worldwide.
- Hypertension is associated with increased cardiovascular mortality and morbidity in all age groups but in the elderly the risk appears to be directly proportional to systolic blood pressure (SBP) and inversely proportional to diastolic blood pressure (DBP).
- There are also independent relationships between hypertension and heart failure, peripheral artery disease and end-stage renal disease.
- Present evidence indicates 50% of patients with hypertension are undiagnosed and only one-tenth have their hypertension treated to target.

Table 9.1 Definition and classification of blood pressure (European Cardiology Society (ECS) guidelines) in mmHg

Category	Systolic	Diastolic
Optimal	<120	<80
Normal	120–129	80–84
High normal	130–139	85–89
Grade 1 Hypertension	140–159	90–99
Grade 2 Hypertension	160–179	100–109
Grade 3 Hypertension	≥180	≥110
Isolated systolic hypertension	≥140	<90

Isolated systolic hypertension (ISH)

- A distinct pathological entity in the elderly arising from reduced vascular compliance resulting in increased SBP and reduced DBP. Age and systolic blood pressure are continuous variables, so arbitrary definitions are used for classification as in Table 9.1.
- The rise in SBP causes left ventricular hypertrophy and the reduction in DBP may compromise coronary blood flow.
- Prevalence increases with age and ISH is the commonest form of hypertension in the elderly.
- Greater cardiovascular risk than diastolic hypertension in the elderly.
- For risk assessment ISH should be graded according to the same systolic blood pressure values indicated for systolic-diastolic hypertension, remembering that low diastolic blood pressure (60–70 mmHg) is an additional risk.

White-coat hypertension/office hypertension

- Diagnosed when office blood pressure is ≥140/90 on at least three occasions while home or 24-hour mean and daytime blood pressures are within normal range (see Diagnosis of hypertension, p. 198).
- More common in elderly people and females.
- Risk appears to be lower than in those with persistent hypertension on both office and home readings but may be greater than in normotensive individuals.

Diagnosis of hypertension

- Blood pressure is characterized by spontaneous variations during the day and between days and months.
- The diagnosis of hypertension is based on multiple measurements, taken on separate occasions over a period of time usually at least two measurements per visit and at least two to three visits.
- If blood pressure is only slightly elevated measurements should be over a period of months (grade 1 and no end-organ damage).
- If the patient has a more marked blood pressure elevation (grade 2) and or evidence of hypertension-related end-organ damage or a high cardiovascular risk profile, repeated measurements should be obtained over shorter periods of time (weeks or days). In particularly severe cases (grade 3 and symptomatic or high cardiovascular risk) the diagnosis can be based on measurements taken at a single visit.
- Blood pressures can be measured by the doctor or nurse in the clinic, by the patient or a relative at home, or automatically over 24 hours (see Box 9.1).

Measurement of blood pressure

- Traditionally blood pressure is measured with a mercury sphygmomanometer, which should be kept in proper working order.
- Non-invasive devices (auscultatory or oscillometric semiautomatic devices) are increasingly used because of the progressive banning of the medical use of mercury. These devices should be validated according to standardized protocols and their accuracy should be checked periodically by comparison with mercury sphygmomanometric values.
- The recommendations for measurement are outlined in Box 9.1.

Box 9.1 Measurement of blood pressure

- Sit patient for several minutes in a quiet room before blood pressure measurements.
- Take at least two measurements spaced by 1–2 minutes, and additional measurements if the these are quite different.
- Use the right size bladder and have the cuff at the heart level.
- Use phase I and V (disappearance) Korotkoff sounds to identify systolic and diastolic blood pressure, respectively.
- Measure blood pressure in both arms at first visit to detect possible differences due to peripheral vascular disease and use the higher value as the reference one.
- Measure blood pressure 1, 3, and 5 minutes after standing in elderly subjects to detect postural hypotension.

Ambulatory blood pressure measurement (ABPM) versus conventional measurement

- Eliminates observer inaccuracy due to systematic error, terminal digit preference, and observer prejudice.
- Allows multiple measurements over the 24-hour period at predetermined times without patient interference.
- More reproducible than office measurements.
- Less subject to the white coat effect.
- Large discrepancies between the blood pressures recorded by the two techniques in elderly patients with ISH but not in normotensive patients.
- ABPMs are lower than office blood pressure measurements – based on current evidence, upper limits for normal for ABPM are set at 125–130/80 (130–135/85 day and 120/70 night) in Europe, but optimum levels have still to be determined and are currently not age related.
- Better predictor of cardiovascular mortality and morbidity than office measurements alone but more data needed in the elderly.

Indications for ABPM

- In case of diagnostic uncertainty, suspect the white coat effect.
- To assess response to treatment, especially if office readings are persistently above target.
- Large variations in blood pressure measurement.
- Suspect resistance to treatment.
- Suspect symptomatic hypotension.

Home blood pressure measurement (HBPM): advantages and current knowledge

- Increasingly popular as more reliable automatic devices are now available.
- Less liable to observer bias and the white coat effect than office blood pressure measurements and can diagnose normal blood pressure with good accuracy.
- HBPMs are lower than office blood pressure measurements – based on current evidence upper limits for normal for HBPM are set at 135/85.
- Correlate well with daytime values of ABPM.
- Correlate better with target organ damage and cardiovascular mortality than office measurements on current evidence but more data needed in the elderly.
- Easier to obtain repeated measurements in elderly patients.
- Facilitates self-management.
- Differences between home and office readings increase with age and height of SBP, and are greater in men and in those not on treatment
- Treatment tend to cause a greater decline in office than home blood pressure readings - this may be related to different types of machine used in the home and office or observer bias; a current trial is addressing this (Home versus Office blood pressure MEasurements: Reduction of Unnecessary treatment Study (HOMERUS) trial)

Recommendations for HBPM
- Use a reliable validated device.
- Follow currently available guidelines and ensure patient education from an experienced nurse or physician.
- In case of diagnostic uncertainty, recommendations at present are duplicate readings twice daily (am and pm) for 3 consecutive days.
- To exclude the white coat effect, which increases with age and is more related to untreated than treated hypertension.
- To assess response to treatment especially if office readings are persistently above target.
- ABPM is still regarded as superior for measuring blood pressure to assess drug efficacy but HBPM is less expensive and less inconvenient for the patient.

Contraindications for using HBPM
- With large arm sizes if no appropriate cuff is available
- With an irregular pulse such as atrial fibrillation (which is common in the elderly) as it is inaccurate
- With vascular stiffening as all validated devices employ the oscillometric technique, which will be unreliable
- Who are unable to follow instructions (e.g., cognitive impairment)
- Where it induces excess anxiety and inappropriate self-modification of treatment.

Available guidelines
A number of guidelines are available for investigation and management of hypertension and all of these emphasize that in addition to the blood pressure measurement other factors need to be taken into account in deciding on treatment thresholds and targets. There factors include:
- Known cardiovascular or peripheral vascular disease
- Diabetes mellitus
- Assessment of 10-year cardiovascular risk (based on Framingham or other risk score) if no previous cardiovascular events
- Evidence of end-organ damage (left ventricular hypertrophy, proteinuria, renal impairment, heart failure, retinopathy)
- Other co-morbidities.

Investigations
Secondary causes of hypertension with the exception of renal parenchymal disease rarely present in the elderly and will not be discussed here. History and physical examination should focus on a search for:
- Aggravating factors, e.g. drugs (non-steroidal anti-inflammatory drugs (NSAIDs), corticosteroids, liquorice, cocaine and amphetamines, erythropoietin, ciclosporin, tacrolimus), diet (excess salt), sedentary lifestyle, obesity and obstructive sleep apnoea
- Evidence of end-organ damage (as above)
- Complications (heart failure, cerebrovascular, and peripheral vascular disease, etc.)
- Co-morbidities (diabetes, atrial fibrillation, falls, cognitive impairment, frailty, and other terminal disease) that may influence treatment.

Routine and recommended investigations in the elderly before treatment are listed in Table 9.2.

Table 9.2 Investigation in the elderly patient with hypertension

Routine:

Fasting plasma glucose

Fasting lipid profile

Serum electrolytes

Serum creatinine and estimated glomerular filtration rate (Modification of Diet in Renal Disease (MDRD) formula)

Haemoglobin and haematocrit

Urinalysis (microalbuminuria via dipstick test and microscopic examination)

12-lead electrocardiogram (ECG; Fig. 9.1)

Recommended:

Echocardiogram

Quantitative proteinuria (if dipstick test positive)

Funduscopy

Glucose tolerance test (if fasting plasma glucose >5.6 mmol/L)

Home and 24-hour ambulatory blood pressure monitoring as outlined above

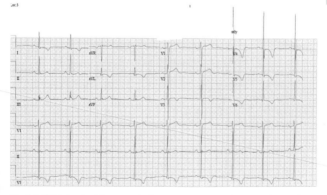

Fig. 9.1 ECG showing left ventricular hypertrophy and repolarization abnormality in a 76-year-old woman with long-standing, difficult-to-control hypertension.

Benefits of treating high blood pressure (randomized controlled trials and meta-analyses)

- Reduced cardiovascular mortality and morbidity with less effect on all-cause mortality.
- Reduction in strokes greater than reduction in coronary events.
- The greater the reduction in blood pressure, the greater the benefit.
- Reduced incidence of heart failure.
- Benefit seen in the elderly and in isolated systolic hypertension.
- Benefit seen across different ethnic groups (Caucasian, Asian, Black, etc.).

Targets

The goal of treatment in the elderly is to reduce cardiovascular risk and other complications such as heart failure and renal failure. This must be balanced against the risk of treatment complications in the elderly, who are more at risk of adverse effects, interactions, and polypharmacy than younger patients. It is also important to address other reversible risk factors identified, including smoking, dyslipidaemia, abdominal obesity, and diabetes, as well as treatment of the raised blood pressure.

Until recently the evidence available for treating patients over 80 years of age with antihypertensive drugs was controversial, but recent evidence suggests a significant benefit in this group also. Treatment should be initiated in this group if indicated according to guidelines (see Chapter 11).

The targets for blood pressure lowering should be similar in the elderly as in younger patients (see Box 9.2) but it is important to remember that blood pressure variability is often greater in the elderly and they are more likely to develop symptomatic hypotension and postural hypotension, so targets may need to be adjusted on an individual basis.

Box 9.2 ECS position statement on treatment goals in hypertensive patients

- Blood pressure should be reduced to at least below 140/90 mmHg, and to lower values, if tolerated, in all hypertensive patients.
- Target blood pressure should be 130/80 mmHg in people with diabetes and in high or very high risk patients, such as those with associated clinical conditions (stroke, myocardial infarction, renal dysfunction, proteinuria).
- Despite use of combination treatment, reducing systolic blood pressure to these levels may be difficult, especially in elderly and diabetic patients, and those with cardiovascular damage.

Treatment

Non-pharmacological

Lifestyle modification does reduce blood pressure and cardiovascular risk and should not be forgotten in the elderly. This includes advice on:

- Weight loss if overweight
- Regular exercise
- Reduced use of salt
- Increased intake of fruit and vegetables
- Reduced alcohol consumption
- Reduced total/saturated fat intake
- Smoking cessation.

Pharmacological

(As recommended by National Institute for Health and Clinical Excellence (NICE; Fig. 9.2) and other guidelines).

- Initial therapy in patients >55 years should be either a calcium channel blocker or a thiazide-type diuretic. However, certain classes of antihypertensive medication are indicated if significant medical conditions coexist, e.g. hypertension with coexisting chronic kidney insufficiency or diabetes is an indication for an angiotensin-converting enzyme (ACE) inhibitor or an angiotensin II receptor (AII) antagonist; a history of myocardial infarction is an indication for B-blockers and ACE inhibitors.
- If initial therapy was with a calcium channel blocker or a thiazide-type diuretic and a second drug is required, add an ACE inhibitor or an AII antagonist if the ACE inhibitor is not tolerated.
- If treatment with three drugs is required, the combination of ACE inhibitor (AII antagonist), calcium channel blocker and thiazide-type diuretic should be used.
- If blood pressure remains uncontrolled on adequate doses of three drugs, consider adding a fourth drug and/or seeking specialist advice.
- If a fourth drug is required, consider:
  - Addition of another diuretic – a loop diuretic or spironolactone (careful monitoring of electrolytes and renal function is essential)
  - Addition of a β-blockers or
  - Addition of a selective α-blocker (e.g. doxazosin), but be aware that it can cause significant postural hypotension in the elderly
  - Combination of ACE and AII antagonist (careful monitoring of renal function is essential)
  - Other vasodilators such as hydralazine or methyldopa may be useful in resistant cases or those with side effects to other drugs; these are usually initiated with specialist advice.
- β-blockers are no longer a preferred initial therapy for hypertension but should be used in patients with ischaemic heart disease or heart failure as indicated for these conditions unless there are contraindications.
- Patients over 80 years should be offered the same treatment as other patients over 55 years, taking account of any co-morbidities and their existing burden of drug use.

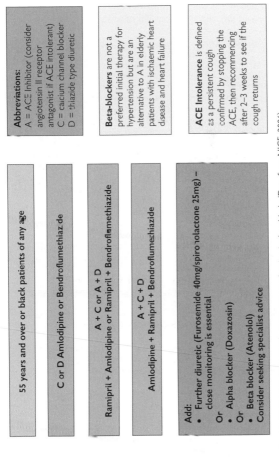

Abbreviations:
A = ACE Inhibitor (consider angiotensin II receptor antagonist if ACE intolerant)
C = cacium channel blocker
D = thiazide type diuretic

Beta-blockers are not a preferred initial therapy for hypertension but are an alternative to A in elderly patients with ischaemic heart disease and heart failure

ACE Intolerance is defined as a persistent cough confirmed by stopping the ACE, then recommencing after 2–3 weeks to see if the cough returns

55 years and over or black patients of any age

C or D Amlodipine or Bendroflumethiazide

A + C or A + D
Ramipril + Amlodipine or Ramipril + Bendroflumethiazide

A + C + D
Amlodipine + Ramipril + Bendroflumethiazide

Add:
- Further diuretic (Furosemide 40mg/spironolactone 25mg) – close monitoring is essential

Or
- Alpha blocker (Doxazosin)

Or
- Beta blocker (Atenolol)
Consider seeking specialist advice

Fig. 9.2 Stepped approach to introducing antihypertensive medication in the elderly (Data from NICE, 2006).

When to refer

Most elderly patients with hypertension can be managed in primary care. Consider referral if:

- Complicated hypertension – associated with significant renal impairment or heart failure
- Failure to respond to three or more antihypertensive drugs
- Significant side effects with treatment
- Concern about the risks versus benefits of treatment.

Follow-up of the elderly patient with hypertension

- Titration to blood pressure control requires frequent visits to modify treatment and check for side effects. In the elderly, this may require home visits if the patient is unable to attend surgery easily.
- Once target blood pressure has been obtained, the frequency of visits can be considerably reduced. Elderly patients should be reviewed at least at 6-monthly intervals to check compliance, side effects including postural hypotension and review the benefits of continuing treatment.
- At follow-up visits check that other reversible risk factors are also controlled (cholesterol, diabetes, smoking, etc.) and reiterate diet and lifestyle advice.
- Annual check of renal function and ECG to assess end-organ damage. In patients on combination of ACE inhibitor and spironolactone or AII receptor blocker monitoring of electrolytes and renal function should be performed 3–6 monthly.
- In general treatment of hypertension should be continued for life but in frail elderly patients reduction or discontinuation of treatment may be appropriate.

Improving compliance and concordance with treatment in the elderly

- Inform the patient of the risk of hypertension and the benefit of effective treatment.
- Provide clear written and oral instructions about treatment.
- Tailor the treatment regimen to patient's lifestyle and needs.
- Simplify treatment by reducing, if possible, the number of daily medications (combination therapy may facilitate this).
- Involve the patient's family or carers in information on disease and treatment plans.
- Make use of self-measurement of blood pressure at home if possible
- Address side effects and alter drug doses or types if necessary.
- Use dossett boxes and blister packs, and medication prompts (e.g. telecare).

Management problems in the elderly hypertensive patient

- Salt restriction is difficult to practise in view of diminished taste sensation and difficulty with shopping for fresh products and cooking.
- Compliance with weight loss and dietary restrictions is often unsuccessful.
- Coexisting diseases preclude certain drug choices.
- Cognitive impairment may affect drug compliance.
- Polypharmacy can lead to drug interactions, drug-related side effects and medication non-concordance.
- Increased risk of inducing symptomatic hypotension, post-prandial hypotension and postural hypotension which may increase risk of falls etc.

Important points to remember

- Hypertension is an important cause of mortality and morbidity in the elderly.
- There is good evidence that treating hypertension even in the very elderly (>80 years) reduces mortality and morbidity from cardiovascular disease.
- The elderly are more susceptible to adverse effects of treatment and symptomatic hypotension.
- Remember that trials include relatively healthy patients and results may not apply to the frail elderly, who may be more at risk of treatment side effects.

Guidelines and recommended reading

British Hypertension Society. Validated blood pressure monitors list. Available from: www.bhsoc.org.

Chobanian AV, Bakris GL, Black HR, Cushman WC, Green LA, Izzo JL Jr, *et al*.; Joint National Committee on Prevention, Detection, Evaluation, and Treatment of High Blood Pressure. National Heart, Lung, and Blood Institute; National High Blood Pressure Education Program Coordinating Committee. (2003) Seventh Report of the Joint National Committee on prevention, detection, evaluation, and treatment of high blood pressure. *Hypertension* **42**:1206–52.

National Institute for Health and Clinical Excellence (2006). Hypertension: management of hypertension in adults in primary care. Clinical guideline 34. London: National Institute for Health and Clinical Excellence. Available from: www.nice.org.uk/cg34.

Task Force for the Management of Arterial Hypertension of the European Society of Hypertension (ESH) and of the European Society of Cardiology (ESC) (2007) 2007 Guidelines for the management of arterial hypertension. Available from: http://www.eshonline.org/Guidelines/ArterialHypertension.aspx.

Key clinical trials in the elderly (see Chapter 11 for more details)

Beckett NS, Peters R, Fletcher AE, Staessen JA, Liu L, Dumitrascu D, *et al*: HYVET Study Group (2008). The **HYVET** (**Hypertension** in the Very Elderly) is the largest clinical trial to date in patients with hypertension over 80 years of age and included 3,854 patients who received slow-release indapamide with the addition of perindopril if required. Significant reductions in all-cause mortality of 21%, cardiovascular events of 34%, and fatal and non-fatal heart failure (64%) were shown. (*N Engl J Med* 2008; **358**:1887–98.)

Gueyffier F, Bulpitt C, Boissel JP, Schron E, Ekbom T, Fagard R, *et al*, INDANA Group (1999) Antihypertensive drugs in very old people: a subgroup meta-analysis of randomised controlled trials. *Lancet* **353**:793–6.

Hansson L, Lindholm LH, Ekbom T, Dahlöf B, Lanke J, Scherstèn B, *et al* (1999). Randomised trail of old (1999) and new antihypertensive drugs in elderly patients: cardiovascular mortality and morbidity in the Swedish trial in old patients with hypertension-2 study (**STOP 2-Hypertension**). *Lancet* **354**:1751–6.

Gong L, Zhang W, Zhu J, Kong D, Pagè V, *et al* (1996). Shanghai trial of nifedipine in the elderly (**STONE**). *J Hypertens* **14**:1237–45.

The **Syst-China Trial** (**Systolic Hypertension in China**). Wang J, Staessen JA, Gong L, Liu L (2000). Chinese trial on isolated systolic hypertension in the elderly. Systolic Hypertension in China (Syst-China Trial). *Arch Intern Med* **160**: 211–220.

Staessen JA, Faggard R, Thijs L, Celis H, Arabidze GG, Birkenhägen WH, *et al* (1997). The **SYS-Eur** (**Systolic Hypertension in Europe**) trial showed that a long-acting dihydropyridine calcium antagonist decreased cardiac endpoints by 26% and stroke by 44% in patients >60 years of age. (*Lancet* 1996; **350**:757–64).

Anon (1992). MRC Working Party (1992) The Medical Research Council trial of treatment of hypertension in older adults: principal results. *BMJ* **304**:405–12.

Anon (1991). The **SHEP (Systolic Hypertension in the Elderly Programme)** included 4736 patients over the age of 65 with SBP >160 and DBP <90 mmHg and showed that diuretic therapy resulted in a 27% reduction in myocardial infarction and coronary heart disease mortality over a 5-year period compared with placebo. (*JAMA* 1991; **265**:3255–64.)

Dahlöf B, Lindholm LH, Hansson L, Scherstén B, Ekbom T, Wester PO (1991). Morbidity and mortality in the Swedish Trial in old patients with hypertension (**STOP-Hypertension**). *Lancet* **338**:1281–5.

Chapter 10

Abdominal aortic aneurysm and peripheral vascular disease

Abdominal aortic aneurysm

- Localized dilatation (>3.5 cm anteroposterior axis) of the aorta related to weakness of the vessel wall.
- M>F (5:1).
- Prevalence increases with age (10% men >80 years).
- Risk factors – smoking, history of peripheral vascular disease (PVD) or ischaemic heart disease, hypertension, genetic predisposition.

Presentation

Incidental finding

Most aneurysms are detected while patients are undergoing examination or investigation for other conditions. Palpation is only sensitive at identifying the presence of an aneurysm if the patient is thin or the aneurysm is >5 cm in size.

Catastrophic rupture

Aneurysm rupture is related to aneurysm size. Many patients in whom aortic aneurysms rupture die outside hospital. The exact incidence is unknown because their sudden death may be attributed to other causes, such as myocardial infarction. Those who do survive long enough to reach hospital, present with abdominal, back, or groin pain and collapse.

Investigation

If an abdominal aortic aneurysm (AAA) is found incidentally, the first-line investigation is abdominal ultrasound. If the patient is considered to be a surgical candidate, they should also have a computed tomography (CT) scan, as this is the most accurate method of investigating whether the aneurysm is extending to the iliac arteries.

In the acute setting (i.e. suspected rupture), the investigation of choice is CT, however, an initial ultrasound scan ('Fast scan') in accident and emergency is increasingly used as a diagnostic tool.

Treatment

Incidental finding

Asymptomatic aneurysm, <5.4 cm

- Ultrasound scan surveillance every 6–12 months.
- Cardiovascular risk management, in particular, good control of blood pressure aiming for 120/80 mmHg if tolerated (see Chapter 9).

Asymptomatic aneurysm, >5.5 cm

- Elective surgical repair – open or endovascular aneurysm repair (EVAR; Table 10.1).
- EVAR often considered if patient unlikely to manage open procedure due to co-morbidities.

Symptomatic but not ruptured

- Repair is indicated as development of pain may indicate impending aneurysm rupture.

Preoperative assessment should include myocardial perfusion imaging to detect unrecognized cardiovascular disease and assessment of physical function (metabolic equivalent of activities of daily living (METs)) – see Chapter 12.

Table 10.1 Comparison of open and endovascular repair of abdominal aortic aneurysms

	Complications	Other
Open repair	Myocardial infarction Pulmonary embolism Mesenteric ischaemia Renal failure Wound infection Graft infection Limb ischaemia Spinal cord ischaemia Perioperative mortality 2–7%	Prosthetic graft sutured from normal proximal to normal distal aorta Prophylactic antibiotics to prevent graft infection
Endovascular aneurysm repair	Endoleak Graft occlusion Graft migration Aortic neck expansion Limb ischaemia Perioperative mortality 0–2%	Transfemoral delivery of covered stent graft into aorta Higher late complication rate (<20%) and need for re-intervention than open repair

AAA rupture

In the acute setting, the decision to perform surgical repair is based on a number of factors:
- Presence of co-morbidities
- Patient's wishes
- Likelihood of survival (e.g. if patient does not respond to initial resuscitation measures, they are unlikely to survive surgery).

The overall mortality is ~90%.

Screening

Screening for AAA may reduce the incidence of rupture. Current UK guidelines advise screening using ultrasound scanning for the following groups:
- Men >60 years with a first-degree relative with AAA
- Male smokers aged 67–75 years.

Screening is still not available in all areas in the UK but should be in the near future as part of the National Screening Committee agenda. There is insufficient evidence to support a screening programme in women.

Prognosis

- AAA will continue to slowly grow and will eventually rupture.
- Repair is delayed until the theoretical risk of rupture exceeds the estimated operative mortality risk.
- Survival at 5 years after intact aneurysm repair is 60–75%.

Peripheral vascular disease

Lower limb disease
- Atherosclerosis of lower limb arteries causes chronic arterial occlusive disease.
- Acute limb ischaemia may occur secondary to emboli or thrombosis on a background of PVD.
- Prevalence increases with age (25% of men aged 80 years).
- M>F (1.4:1).
- Risk factors include smoking, diabetes, hypertension and dyslipidaemia.
- Often coexists with coronary artery disease and/or carotid artery disease – management of PVD provides an opportunity for secondary prevention of cardiovascular events, which must not be missed as many of these patients will die from cardiovascular disease.
- PVD is a chronic disease that can be controlled but not cured.

Presentation
History
- Intermittent claudication – pain or weakness on walking which is relieved by rest and reoccurs on walking again. Claudication pain most commonly affects calf, but may also affect buttocks, hips, thighs or inferior back muscles if there is atherosclerotic disease in the distal aorta and iliac arteries. Only 50% of elderly patients with PVD are symptomatic because:
  - Co-morbidities (e.g. osteoarthritis or chronic obstructive pulmonary disease (COPD)) limit exertion before muscle ischaemia is induced
  - Atypical symptoms are not recognized as claudication
  - Development of sufficient collateral circulation avoids ongoing symptoms.
- Differential diagnoses include spinal stenosis, osteoarthritis, and venous claudication.
- Arterial ulceration – chronic arterial insufficiency may result in ulcers at the ankle, leg, or heel.
- Erectile dysfunction.
- Rest pain – due to critical ischaemia i.e. if the blood flow is insufficient to meet the needs of lower limb tissues at rest. This is usually worse at night and relieved by hanging legs out of bed (to increase blood flow to affected areas).
- Gangrene – ischaemic infarction of toes, associated with critical limb ischaemia.
- Pain, paralysis, paraesthesia, pallor, pulselessness – the five 'Ps' associated with acute limb ischaemia secondary to a sudden decrease in limb perfusion.

Examination
- Arterial pulses – may be decreased or absent.
- Cold feet.
- Arterial ulceration.
- Signs of critical ischaemia – muscle atrophy, hair loss over affected area, thickened toenails, pale extremities, shiny skin.
- Ankle brachial pressure index (ABPI; Table 10.2) – is the measurement of ankle (dorsalis pedis or posterior tibial) and brachial systolic pressures using hand-held Doppler. ABPI <0.9 is 95% sensitive for diagnosis of PVD.

NB ABPI may not be accurate in patients with non-compressible arteries (e.g. diabetic patients).

Table 10.2 The ankle brachial pressure index (ABPI)*

ABPI	Symptoms
0.9–1.2	Normal
0.6–0.9	Mild to moderate intermittent claudication
0.4–0.6	Severe intermittent claudication
0.25–0.4	Rest pain, tissue loss (ulcers, gangrene)

*Highest ankle systolic pressure/highest brachial systolic pressure.

Investigation

The decision to investigate further should involve consideration of treatment options and should occur after medical management has been commenced unless there is critical ischaemia.

- Duplex ultrasound – to assess location and degree of stenosis. Less accurate in tortuous, calcified vessels or prosthetic grafts.
- Angiography – digital subtraction arteriography. Contraindications include allergy to contrast and renal failure (Fig. 10.1).
- CT angiography/magnetic resonance angiography – less sensitive than traditional angiography but useful for imaging other pathologies associated with PVD, e.g. aneurysms.

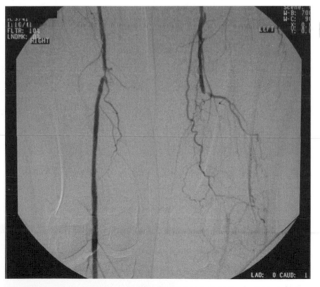

Fig. 10.1 Angiogram showing occlusion of the left superficial femoral artery and stenosis of the right superficial femoral artery in 75-year-old man presenting with progressive and limiting claudication. He had a good response to angioplasty.

Differential diagnosis

Conditions with similar presentation to PVD are listed in Table 10.3.

Table 10.3 Differential diagnosis of peripheral vascular disease

Condition	Typical symptoms
Venous claudication	Tight bursting pain affecting whole leg but worse in thigh and groin. Occurs during walking, subsides slowly with rest, is relieved by limb elevation. Often remote history of iliofemoral deep vein thrombosis
Neurogenic claudication	Weakness > pain. Felt in buttock, thigh and hip in a dermatomal distribution. Starts on walking or after standing and relieved by rest and lumbar spinal flexion (sitting or stooping). Usually there is a history of back pain
Osteoarthritis hip	Aching pain in hip, which comes on after walking a variable distance and is not quickly relieved by rest
Chronic compartment syndrome	Tight bursting pain in calf muscles, which comes on after a lot of exercise. Subsides slowly and relief is speeded by elevation. Often in muscular athletes, so rare in the elderly

Treatment

For all treatments, the risks and benefits should be considered. Surgical treatments carry significant risk to life and patients may prefer to live with the disability. Also, treating PVD surgically may unmask other function limiting co-morbidities (e.g. COPD, angina).

For all patients

- Modify risk factors, e.g. stop smoking, optimize blood pressure and diabetic control, treat dyslipidaemia.
- Antiplatelet therapy with aspirin 75 mg od (or clopidogrel 75 mg od if aspirin intolerant – aspirin intolerance is defined as hypersensitivity to aspirin or severe dyspepsia induced by low-dose aspirin) unless contraindicated. Based on subgroup analysis of the CAPRIE (Clopidogrel versus Aspirin in Patients at Risk of Ischaemic Events) trial, clopidogrel appeared to be superior to aspirin in preventing cardiovascular events in patients with PVD but aspirin remains first line at present. On present evidence there is no indication for dual antiplatelet therapy in PVD, but it may be indicated for coexistent coronary heart disease (CHD; see Chapter 3).
- Encourage exercise; consider an exercise rehabilitation programme if there is one available locally.
- Avoid trauma to feet and lower limbs (high risk of ulceration and poor wound healing). Assistance with toe nail clipping and application of topical emollients reduces the risk of injury or infection. Referral to podiatry services is especially important in elderly patients who may have difficulties with good foot care.
- Consider β-blockers, especially if there is coexistent coronary artery disease and in patients being considered for operative intervention (see Chapter 12). Meta-analysis shows no deterioration in claudication

or walking distance in patients with PVD treated with B-blockers but they should be used with caution and only with specialist advice in patients with critical ischaemia.

- Consider angiotensin-converting enzyme (ACE) inhibitor therapy if patient is hypertensive and or diabetic. ACE inhibitors should be introduced cautiously with careful monitoring of renal function as patients may have renovascular disease. If renal function deteriorates significantly (creatinine more than doubles), specialist advice should be sought.

Medical management

Only cilostazol and naftidrofuryl (Table 10.4) have been shown to improve walking distance in patients with PVD and intermittent claudication.

Table 10.4 Cilostazol and naftidrofuryl

	Effects	Adverse effects	Contraindications
Cilostazol	Vasodilator, antiplatelet	Gastrointestinal disturbance, tachycardia, arrhythmia, chest pain, oedema, dizziness, rash, rhinitis, pruritus	Heart failure (ejection fraction <40%), predisposition to bleeding (e.g. peptic ulcer, haemorrhagic stroke), renal impairment
Naftidrofuryl	Vasodilator	Nausea, epigastric pain, rash, hepatitis, hepatic failure	

Revascularization

Transluminal angioplasty or bypass surgery. Consider if incapacitating claudication, limb salvage (e.g. rest pain, non-healing ulcers, gangrene) or vasculogenic impotence. Patients considered for revascularization procedures should have been able to walk prior to the incident of critical ischaemia, be able to withstand surgery and have a life expectancy of >1 year.

Angioplasty ± stent

For disease localized to vessel segment <10 cm long in iliac or femoral artery.

Bypass surgery

For extensive, diffuse, or multilevel disease.

Guidelines for when to refer to specialist

Most patients with PVD can be managed in primary care. Indications for specialist referral are listed in Box 10.1 and will depend on local expertise and availability of non-invasive tests in the community.

> **Box 10.1 Indications for specialist referral**
>
> - Critical limb ischaemia – requires urgent referral.
> - Limiting symptoms and objective evidence of vascular disease.
> - Unsure of diagnosis or lack of access to non-invasive investigation.
> - Unable to control risk factors to recommended targets.

Acute limb ischaemia

- Treatment options depend on whether limb is viable or not, and the pre-morbid function of the patient.
- Amputation considered if life expectancy is low (i.e. rapid symptomatic relief but resulting loss of function), tissue loss has exceeded point of salvage, function is affected by co-morbidities such that limb salvage has no additional benefit or if revascularization surgery considered too risky.
- If the limb is viable, initial treatment is localized – intra-arterial thrombolysis with alteplase. If a patient continues to have symptoms, they should undergo revascularization.

Prognosis

- Intermittent claudication associated with ~1% risk of limb loss per year and 6–10% risk of requiring intervention for critical ischaemia.
- In patients with critical limb ischaemia, there is a 1-year mortality of 25–45%.
- Patients with PVD have a high risk of cardiovascular morbidity and mortality so good control of risk factors is essential to reduce cardiovascular events.

Guidelines and recommended reading

http://bestpractice.bmj.com/best-practice/monograph/431.html (and /145.html)

Cosford PA, Leng GC (2007) Screening for abdominal aortic aneurysm. *Cochrane Database Syst Rev* CD002945 Issue 2. Available from: www.cochrane.org.

Hirsch AT, Haskal ZJ, Hertzer NR, Bakal CW, Creager MA, Halperin JL, *et al.* (2005) Practice Guidelines for the management of patients with peripheral arterial disease (lower extremity, renal, mesenteric, and abdominal aortic): a collaborative report from the American Association for Vascular Surgery/Society for Vascular Surgery, Society for Cardiovascular Angiography and Interventions, Society for Vascular Medicine and Biology, Society of Interventional Radiology, and the ACC/AHA Task Force on Practice Guidelines (Writing Committee to Develop Guidelines for the Management of Patients With Peripheral Arterial Disease): endorsed by the American Association of Cardiovascular and Pulmonary Rehabilitation; National Heart, Lung, and Blood Institute; Society for Vascular Nursing; TransAtlantic Inter-Society Consensus; and Vascular Disease Foundation. *Circulation* **113**:e463–654.

National Institute for Health and Clinical Excellence (2006) Stent-graft placement in abdominal aortic aneurysm. Interventional procedure guidance 163. London: National Institute for Health and Clinical Excellence. Available from: www.nice.org.uk/ipg163

Pathy J, Sinclair AJ, Morley JE (eds) (2006) *Principles and practice of geriatric medicine.* 4th edn. Chichester: John Wiley.

Scottish Intercollegiate Guidelines Network (2006) Diagonis and management of peripheral arterial disease. Clinical guideline 89. Edinburgh: Scottish Intercollegiate Guidelines Network. Available from: http://www.sign.ac.uk/guidelines/fulltext/89/index.html ISBN 1899893547.

Chapter 11

Major clinical trials and the elderly

Introduction

- Evidence from well-conducted, randomized controlled trials is an important guide to clinical management, and in cardiology we are fortunate to have much such evidence.
- However, the elderly, who have the greatest burden of cardiovascular disease, have largely been excluded from these trials, and this has contributed to ageism in treating elderly patients with cardiovascular disease.
- In this chapter we discuss some of the trials that have been conducted mainly (but not all) in the elderly to demonstrate that trials in the elderly are feasible and that elderly people gain considerable benefits from treatment both in terms of quality and quantity of life. We have restricted ourselves to some of the important trials we feel have significantly affected management.
- It is important that future clinical trials must include the elderly.

Trials in ischaemic heart disease

TIME (Trial of Invasive versus Medical therapy in Elderly Patients)

Reference: TIME Investigators (2001) Trial of Invasive versus Medical therapy in Elderly patients with chronic symptomatic coronary artery disease: a randomised trial, *Lancet* **358**:951–7.

Study question: Which treatment improves the quality of life (QoL) and outcome of elderly patients with angina more, invasive therapy or medical management?

Short answer: Invasive therapy, although the initial risks are higher.

Study population: Patients aged >75 treated with at least 2 anti-anginal drugs and still experiencing symptoms. Exclusion criteria included recent MI, concomitant valvular/other heart disease, life-limiting co-morbid disease, severe renal failure, and heart failure.

Method: Participants randomized into 2 treatment groups; invasive therapy (coronary angiography ± revascularization or PCI if feasible) and optimized medical therapy (addition of further anti-anginal medication or dose increase (>55%) in current medication). Endpoints at 6 and 12 months, including QoL, relief from angina, and freedom from major adverse clinical events (e.g. death, MI, hospitalization for refractory angina or ACS).

Results: 301 patients randomized, 153 to invasive therapy, 148 to optimized medical therapy. In invasive group, 52% received PCI, 20% underwent CABG, remaining 28% had medical management only. In medical therapy group, 55 patients required invasive therapy for uncontrollable symptoms. QoL improved in both groups, but improvement was greater after revascularization. Fewer major adverse cardiac events occurred in the invasive group (29 vs 72), although there was a small excess early mortality when compared with medical therapy.

Conclusion: Elderly patients with persistent angina despite medication have better symptom control and QoL after revascularization compared with optimized medical therapy.

Impact on management of elderly patients: Elderly patients with chronic angina refractory to medication should be referred for consideration of invasive therapy (e.g. PCI or CABG).

TIME: 4-year follow-up

Reference: Pfisterer M; Trial of Invasive versus Medical therapy in Elderly patients Investigators (2004) Long-term outcome in elderly patients with chronic angina managed invasively versus by optimized medical therapy. Four-year follow-up of the randomized trial of invasive versus medical therapy in older patients (TIME). *Circulation* **110**:1213–18.

Study question: What were the longer term outcomes of the TIME participants?

Short answer: Long-term survival was the same in both groups but those who were revascularized in the first year had better survival rates (regardless of their initial group).

Study population: Survivors of the 1-year TIME trial; 137 in invasive therapy group, 139 in medical therapy group.

Method: Participants were followed up by questionnaire <3 years after the end of the initial trial. Endpoints were death, hospitalizations for cardiac events, QoL , angina severity and anti-anginal drug use.

Results: There was no significant difference in death rate between the 2 groups (29.4% for invasive group, 27.0% for medical group). Revascularization within the first year resulted in better long-term survival. Cardiac re-hospitalizations less frequent in the invasive therapy group (12% vs 45%). QoL improvements maintained in both groups.

Conclusion: Invasive therapy associated with early symptom relief and improvement in wellbeing but related procedural risks. Medical therapy associated with greater number of medications and higher re-hospitalization rate but similar mortality.

Impact on management of elderly patients: Elderly patients with chronic angina should be considered for invasive therapy if symptoms persist, but medical therapy is a valid option.

APPROACH (Alberta Provincial Project for Outcomes Assessment in Coronary Heart disease)

References: Graham MM, Ghali WA, Faris PD, Galbraith PD, Norris CM, Knudtson ML; Alberta Provincial Project for Outcomes Assessment in Coronary Heart Disease (APPROACH) Investigators. Survival after coronary revascularization in the elderly (2002) *Circulation* **105**:2378–84; and Graham MM, Norris CM, Galbraith PD, Knudtson ML, Ghali WA; APPROACH Investigators (2006) Quality of life after coronary revascularization in the elderly. *Eur Heart J* **27**:1690–8.

Study question: What happens to patients after they have had cardiac catheterization and do different treatments significantly affect mortality and QoL?

Short answer: Patients treated with invasive therapy tend to have better survival and QoL.

Study population: All patients on the Alberta Provincial Project for Outcomes Assessment in Coronary Heart disease database, i.e. all patients in Alberta (Canada) undergoing cardiac catheterization between 1995 and 1998.

Method: Database reviewed regarding therapeutic interventions (performed within 1 year) and survival of patients post catheterization. Patients also sent a health status questionnaire (Seattle Angina Questionnaire) 1, 3, and 5 years post initial catheterization.

Results: Elderly patients analysed in 2 main groups: 70–79 years and ≥80 years. Each group had 3 subgroups depending on intervention – CABG, PCI, or medical therapy. 5198 patients in 70–79 group and 983 ≥80 years. Survival at 4 years post catheterization was 87.3% (CABG), 83.9% (PCI), 79.1% (medical therapy) in 70–79 years group and 77.4%, 71.6%, and 60.3%, respectively, in those ≥80. At 1 year, patients aged 70–79 treated with CABG or PCI had significantly better SAQ scores compared with medical therapy group. Those ≥80 years had significantly better scores if treated with CABG. Findings persisted at 3 years.

Conclusion: Survival and QoL improved by revascularization procedures. Results should be interpreted with caution as patients in medical therapy group had more co-morbidities.

Impact on management of elderly patients: Elderly patients with ischaemic heart disease should be considered for revascularization (PCI or CABG).

Trials in heart failure

SENIORS (Study of Effects of Nebivolol Intervention on Outcomes and Rehospitalisation in Seniors with heart failure)

Reference: Flather MD, Shibata MC, Coats AJ, Van Veldhuisen DJ, Parkhomenko A, *et al.*; SENIORS Investigators (2005) Randomized trial to determine the effect of nebivolol on mortality and cardiovascular hospital admission in elderly patients with heart failure (SENIORS) *Eur Heart J* **26**:215–25.

Study question: Does nebivolol reduce mortality and morbidity of elderly patients with heart failure?

Short answer: Yes.

Study population: Patients aged ≥70 years with history of heart failure (EF ≤35% or hospital admission for heart failure within previous year). Exclusion criteria included new (<6 weeks) drug therapy for heart failure, heart failure due to uncorrected valvular disease, contraindication/intolerance to β-blocker and significant hepatic or renal dysfunction.

Method: Double-blind, placebo-controlled trial. Target dose of nebivolol was 10 mg od. Placebo group received matching placebos. Participants reviewed 3-monthly for mean 21 months. Primary outcome was composite of all-cause mortality or cardiovascular hospital admission (time to first event). Secondary outcomes included cardiovascular mortality and hospital admissions and functional capacity (NYHA class assessment).

Results: 2128 patients randomized, 1067 received nebivolol, 1061 received placebo. Mean age was 76 years. Nebivolol group had significantly lower rate of death or cardiovascular admission (31.1% vs 35.3%, hazard ratio 0.86, p = 0.039). There was no significant difference in all-cause mortality or all-cause hospitalization. Beneficial effects not apparent until participants had been treated for 6 months.

Conclusion: Treating elderly patients with heart failure with nebivolol reduces the composite risk of all-cause mortality or cardiovascular hospital admission compared with placebo.

Impact on management of elderly patients: Consider adding nebivolol to treatment regimen of elderly heart failure patients if tolerated.

ELITE (Evaluation of Losartan In The Elderly)

Reference: Pitt B, Segal R, Martinez FA, Meurers G, Cowley AJ, Thomas I, et al. (1997) Randomized trial of losartan vs captopril in patients over 65 with heart failure: Evaluation of Losartan In The Elderly Study, ELITE. *Lancet* **349**:747–52.

Study question: How does losartan compare with captopril in the treatment of older heart failure patients?

Short answer: About the same in efficacy but losartan better tolerated.

Study population: Patients aged >65 with symptomatic heart failure (NYHA II–IV), decreased ejection fraction (<40%) and no history of prior ACE inhibitor therapy. Exclusion criteria included hypotension (systolic BP <90 mmHg), contraindications to vasodilator therapy, recent MI (<72 hours), serum creatinine >220 µmol/l, significant obstructive valve disease, constrictive pericarditis, symptomatic ventricular/supraventricular arrhythmias.

Method: Participants randomized to 48 weeks of therapy, with captopril (50 mg tds) and placebo or losartan (50 mg od) and placebo. Weekly clinical assessments until on maximum tolerated dose then 3 monthly. Endpoints included renal dysfunction (creatinine increase >10%), mortality and hospitalizations for heart failure, cough, and hypotension-related symptoms.

Results: 722 patients randomized; 352 losartan and 370 captopril. Persisting rise in creatinine of >10% occurred in both groups at same rate (10.5%). All cause mortality lower in losartan group (4.8% vs 8.7%, p = 0.035), largely due to reduction in cardiac deaths. No difference between the 2 groups with regard to frequency of hospitalizations for heart failure or improvement in NYHA class. More patients in captopril group (20.8%) discontinued therapy due to side effects (cough, hyperkalaemia, worsening heart failure, rash, hypotension). In the losartan group 12.2% stopped therapy due to hypotension and renal dysfunction.

Conclusion: Losartan is as efficacious as captopril in treating older patients with heart failure and is better tolerated with the added benefit of small reduction in risk of mortality.

Impact on management of elderly patients: Losartan is a safe alternative to captopril in elderly patients.

Trials in heart failure with preserved systolic function (diastolic heart failure)

PEP-CHF (Perindopril in Elderly People with Chronic Heart Failure)

Reference: Cleland JG, Tendera M, Adamus J, Freemantle N, Polonski L, Taylor J; PEP-CHF Investigators (2006) The perindopril in elderly people with chronic heart failure (PEP-CHF) study. *Eur Heart J* **27**:2338–45.

Study question: Does perindopril improve outcome in patients with heart failure and echocardiogram evidence of diastolic dysfunction?

Short answer: Probably yes.

Study population: Patients aged ≥70 years with a diagnosis of heart failure, treated with diuretics and echocardiogram suggesting diastolic dysfunction. Patients with LV systolic dysfunction or valve disease were excluded.

Method: Randomized, double-blind trial, comparing placebo with perindopril, 4 mg/day. The primary endpoint was a composite of all-cause mortality and unplanned heart failure related hospitalization with a minimum follow-up of 1 year.

Results: 850 patients were randomized with mean age 76 ± 5 years. 55% were female. Median follow-up was 2.1 years. Many patients withdrew from perindopril (28%) and placebo (26%) after 1 year and started taking open-label ACE-inhibitors which reduced the power of the study. 107 patients assigned to placebo and 100 assigned to perindopril reached the primary endpoint (HR 0.919; 95% CI 0.700 to 1.208; p = 0.545). By 1 year, reductions in the primary outcome (HR 0.692; 95% CI 0.474 to 1.010; p = 0.055) and hospitalization for heart failure (HR 0.628; 95% CI 0.408 to 0.966; p = 0.033) were observed and functional class (p <0.030) and 6-minute walk distance (p = 0.011) improved in those assigned to perindopril.

Conclusion: The effects of perindopril on long-term morbidity and mortality are uncertain. Improved symptoms, exercise capacity, and fewer hospitalizations for heart failure in the first year were observed, suggesting perindopril may be of benefit in this patient population.

Impact on management of elderly patients: Perindopril should be considered in elderly patients with symptoms of heart failure and preserved systolic function.

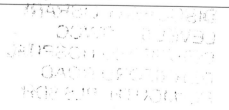

CHARM-Preserved (Candesartan in patients with heart failure and preserved systolic function)

Reference: Yusuf S, Pfeffer MA, Swedberg K, Gvanger CB, Held P, McMuray JJ et al. CHARM Investigators and Committees. (2003) Effects of candesartan in patients with chronic heart failure and preserved systolic function: the CHARM-Preserved Trial. *Lancet* **362** 777–81.

Study question: Does candesartan reduce mortality and morbidity in patients with chronic heart failure and preserved systolic function?

Short answer: Yes.

Study population: Patients with symptomatic chronic heart failure were recruited into 1 of 3 specific studies depending on LVEF and tolerability to ACE inhibitor: group 1, patients with LVEF <40% and intolerant of ACE inhibitors (CHARM-Alternative); group 2, patients with LVEF <40% treated with an ACE inhibitor (CHARM-Added); and group 3, patients with preserved systolic function and not on ACE inhibitor treatment (CHARM-Preserved).

Method: Parallel, randomized, double-blind, controlled clinical trials comparing candesartan titrated to 32 mg daily with placebo in the three groups. The primary outcome for the whole study was all-cause mortality and for all the component trials was cardiovascular death or hospital admission for CHF.

Results: Candesartan was generally well tolerated and significantly reduced cardiovascular deaths and hospital admissions for heart failure in the whole study (all 3 groups). 3023 patients were enrolled in group 3 and followed up for at least 2 years. 22% in the candesartan and 24% in the placebo group experienced the primary outcome (unadjusted HR 0.89; 95% CI 0.77 to 1.03; p = 0.118; covariate adjusted 0.86 (0.74 to 1.0; p = 0.051). Cardiovascular death did not differ between groups, but fewer patients in the candesartan group than in the placebo group were admitted to hospital for CHF (230 vs 279; p = 0.017) and frequency of admissions was also reduced.

Conclusion: Candesartan reduces admissions for CHF in patients with heart failure and LVEF >40%.

Impact on management of elderly patients: Candesartan is beneficial in patients with symptomatic heart failure and preserved systolic function. In patients with reduced EF, candesartan is a useful alternative in patients intolerant to ACE and as add on in patients who have persistent symptoms on ACE (see *Lancet* (2003) **326**:759–766).

I-Preserve (Irbesartan in patients with heart failure and preserved EF)

Reference: Massie BM, Carson PE, McMurray JJ, Komajda M, McKelvie R, Zile MR, *et al.*; I-PRESERVE Investigators (2008) Irbesartan in patients with heart failure and preserved ejection fraction. *N Engl J Med* **359**:2456–67.

Study question: To evaluate the effect of irbesartan on mortality and cardiovascular morbidity in patients with heart failure and preserved ejection fraction.

Short answer: No benefit.

Study population: 4128 patients aged ≥60 years, in NYHA Class II–IV, and with an EF ≥45%. Mean age was 72 ± 7 years and 60% were female. All patients had a recent hospitalization for heart failure or corroborative evidence of it, such as pulmonary congestion or LVH.

Method: Randomized to receive irbesartan 300 mg/day or placebo and followed-up for a median of 49.5 months. The primary composite outcome was death from any cause or hospitalization for cardiovascular cause (heart failure, MI, unstable angina, arrhythmia, or stroke). Secondary outcomes were death from heart failure, hospitalization for heart failure, death from any cause and cardiovascular causes, and quality of life.

Results: No difference in the primary outcome between irbesartan (36%) and placebo (37%). No difference in any of the secondary outcomes including hospitalization for heart failure.

Conclusion: Irbesartan did not improve the outcomes of patients with heart failure and preserved LVEF. This is in contrast to the PEP-CHF (p. 230) and Charm-Preserved (p. 231) trials.

Impact on management of elderly patients: In contrast to candesartan there is no evidence that irbesartan improves symptoms or reduces admissions in patients with heart failure and preserved systolic function. The reasons for this difference are unclear at present.

Hong Kong Diastolic Heart Failure Study

Reference: Yip GW, Wang M, Wang T, Chan S, Fung JW, Yeung L, et al. (2008) The Hong Kong Diastolic Heart Failure Study: a randomized controlled trial of diuretics, irbesartan and ramipril on quality of life, exercise capacity, left ventricular global and regional function in heart failure with a normal ejection fraction. *Heart* **94**:573–80.

Study question: Does renin-angiotensin system blockade in addition to diuretics affect quality of life or LV function in patients with heart failure and normal EF?

Short answer: No significant benefit.

Study population: 150 patients with heart failure and EF >45%. Mean age was 74 ± 8 and >60% female.

Method: Randomized to: group 1, diuretics alone; group 2, diuretics + irbesartan; and group 3, diuretics + ramipril. QoL, 6-minute walk test (6MWT) and Doppler echocardiography at baseline, 12, 24 and 52 weeks.

Results: The QoL score improved similarly in all three groups by 52 weeks (46%, 51%, and 50% respectively). No significant effect on 6MWT. Recurrent hospitalization rates were equal in all groups (9–12% in 1 year). At 1 year, LV dimensions or EF did not change. Systolic and diastolic blood pressures were lowered in all three groups. NT-pro-BNP levels were raised at baseline and fell significantly in the irbesartan and ramipril groups only.

Conclusion: In elderly patients with heart failure and normal LVEF, diuretic therapy significantly improved symptoms and neither irbesartan nor ramipril had a significant additional effect. Small study so interpret with caution.

Impact on management of elderly patients: Diuretics improve symptoms in patients with heart failure and preserved LVEF so useful as first-line therapy.

SWEDIC Study (Swedish Doppler-echocardiographic study)

Reference: Bergström A, Andersson B, Edner M, Nylander E, Persson H, Dahlström U (2004) Effect of carvedilol on diastolic function in patients with diastolic heart failure and preserved systolic function. Results of the Swedish Doppler echocardiographic study. *Eur J Heart Failure* **6**:453–61.

Study question: Does carvedilol improve diastolic function in patients with heart failure and preserved systolic function?

Short answer: Probably yes.

Study population: 113 patients with heart failure and preserved systolic function and abnormal diastolic function treated with conventional therapy. Mean age 66 (48–84) years.

Method: Double-blind, placebo-controlled trial. Follow-up for 6 months after up-titration. The primary endpoint was improved diastolic function as determined by changes in mitral flow velocities (E:A ratio). Secondary endpoints included all-cause mortality, cardiovascular mortality, cardiovascular admissions, and heart failure admissions.

Results: There was no effect on the primary endpoint. A trend towards a better effect in carvedilol-treated patients was noticed in patients with heart rates above 71 bpm. At the end of the study, there was a statistically significant improvement in E:A ratio in patients treated with carvedilol (0.72 to 0.83) versus placebo (0.71 to 0.76), $p<0.05$.

Conclusion: Treatment with carvedilol resulted in a significant improvement in E:A ratio in patients with heart failure due to a LV dysfunction. E:A ratio was found to be the most useful variable to identify diastolic dysfunction in this patient population. This is a small study so interpret with caution.

Impact on management of elderly patients: Carvedilol may be beneficial in patients with heart failure and diastolic dysfunction on echo if heart rate is >71 bpm.

Trials in pacing

ADEPT (Advanced Elements of Pacing Randomised Controlled Trial)

Reference: Lamas GA, Knight JD, Sweeney MO, Mianulli M, Jorapur V, Khalighi K, *et al.* (2007) Impact of rate-modulated pacing on quality of life and exercise capacity – evidence from the Advanced Elements of Pacing Randomised Controlled Trial (ADEPT). *Heart Rhythm* **4**:1133–5.

Study question: Does dual-chamber rate modulated pacing improve quality of life compared with dual-chamber pacing alone?

Short answer: No.

Study population: 872 patients with mean age 71, 64% male with standard indication for dual-chamber pacing (64% had sinus node dysfunction.

Method: Single-blind, randomized controlled trial. Patients were randomized in a factorial design to (1) dual-chamber rate-modulated pacing (DDDR) versus dual-chamber pacing (DDD). The primary endpoint was the score on the Specific Activity Scale, an activity-based cardiovascular disease-specific instrument at 1 year. Secondary endpoints included 6-month treadmill time and additional cardiovascular disease-specific, and generic health-related QoL instruments at 1 year.

Results: At 6 months, patients with rate modulation had a higher peak exercise heart rate (rate modulation 113.3 ± 19.6, no rate modulation 101.1 ± 21.1; p<0.0001) but total exercise time was not different between groups. At 1 year, there were no significant differences between groups with respect to Specific Activity Scale or the secondary QoL endpoints.

Conclusion: Rate modulation is ineffective in improving the functional status or QoL of patients with a bradycardia indication for dual chamber pacing.

Impact on management of elderly patients: No evidence that rate responsive pacing is better than dual chamber pacing.

UKPACE (Single chamber versus dual chamber pacing for atrioventricular block)

Reference: Toff WD, Camm AJ, Skehan JD; United Kingdom Pacing and Cardiovascular Events Trial Investigators (2005) Single-chamber versus dual-chamber pacing for high grade atrioventricular block. *N Engl J Med* **353**:145–55.

Study question: Is dual chamber pacing better than single chamber pacing in elderly patients with atrioventricular block?

Short answer: No difference in mortality at 5 years or cardiovascular events at 3 years.

Study population: Elderly patients with high-grade atrioventricular block, mean age 80 ± 6, 57% male.

Method: Multicentre, randomized, parallel-group trial of 2021 patients 70 years of age or older undergoing first pacemaker implant for high-grade atrioventricular block. Randomly assigned to receive a single chamber ventricular pacemaker (1009 patients) or a dual chamber pacemaker (1012 patients). In the single chamber group, patients were randomly assigned to receive either fixed-rate pacing (504 patients) or rate-adaptive pacing (505 patients). The primary outcome was death from all causes. Secondary outcomes included atrial fibrillation, heart failure, and a composite of stroke, TIA, or other thrombo-embolism.

Results: Median follow-up period was 4.6 years for mortality and 3 years for other cardiovascular events. Mean annual mortality rate was 7.2% in the single chamber group and 7.4% in the dual chamber group (HR 0.96; 0.83–1.11). There were no significant differences between the groups in the rates of atrial fibrillation, heart failure, or the composite of stroke, TIA, or other thrombo-embolism. 3.1% crossed over from single to dual chamber pacing.

Conclusion: In elderly patients with high-grade atrioventricular block, the pacing mode does not influence mortality during the first 5 years or the incidence of cardiovascular events during the first 3 years after implantation of a pacemaker.

Impact on management of elderly patients: In elderly patients with high-grade atrioventricular block the mode of pacing should be decided on an individual basis.

CTOPP (Trial of physiological pacing versus ventricular pacing)

Reference: Connolly SJ, Kerr CR, Gent M, Roberts RS, Yusuf S, Gillis AM, *et al.* (2000) Effects of physiologic pacing versus ventricular pacing on the risk of stroke and death due to cardiovascular causes. Canadian Trial of Physiologic Pacing Investigators. *N Engl J Med* **342**:1385–91; and Kerr CR, Connolly SJ, Abdollah H, Roberts RS, Gent M, Yusuf S, *et al.* (2004) Canadian Trial of Physiological Pacing: Effects of physiological pacing during long-term follow-up. *Circulation* **109**:357–62.

Study question: Is physiological pacing (dual chamber or atrial) superior to ventricular pacing?

Short answer: No – except for development of atrial fibrillation.

Study population: Patients scheduled for a first implantation of a pacemaker to treat symptomatic bradycardia. Mean age was 73 ± 10 years and 59% were male. Patients with atrial fibrillation were excluded.

Method: 1471 were randomly assigned patients to receive a ventricular pacemaker and 1094 a physiologic pacemaker and followed for an average of 3 years and 6 years in the long-term follow-up study. The primary outcome was stroke or death due to cardiovascular causes. Secondary outcomes were death from any cause, atrial fibrillation, and hospitalization for heart failure.

Results: There was no significant difference in the annual rate of stroke or death due to cardiovascular causes between the ventricular pacing and physiological pacing groups at 3 or 6 years (5.5 vs 4.9% at 3 years and 6.1% vs 5.5% at 6 years). The annual rate of atrial fibrillation was significantly lower among the patients in the physiological pacing group (5.3% vs 6.6% at 3 years, relative risk of reduction of 18.0%, p = 0.05) at 3 years and at 6 years (relative risk reduction of 20.1%, p = 0.009). All-cause mortality and hospitalization for heart failure were not significantly different. Perioperative complications were more common with physiological pacing than with ventricular pacing (9.0% vs 3.8%, p<0.001).

Conclusion: Physiologic pacing provides little benefit over ventricular pacing for the prevention of stroke or death due to cardiovascular causes.

Impact on management of elderly patients: In elderly patients requiring pacing for symptomatic bradycardia the mode of pacing should be decided on an individual basis.

MOST (Mode selection trial in sinus node dysfunction)

Reference: Lamas GA, Lee K, Sweeney M, Leon A, Yee R, Ellenbogan K, *et al.* (2002) Mode selection trial in sinus node dysfunction. *Lancet* **346**:1854–62.

Study question: Ventricular pacing or dual chamber pacing for sinus node dysfunction. Which is better?

Short answer: Dual chamber pacing is better.

Study population: The indication for pacing was sinus node dysfunction and 21% also had atrioventricular block. The median age was 74 (68–80) years and 48% were female.

Method: 2010 patients with sinus node dysfunction randomly assigned to dual chamber pacing (1014 patients) or ventricular pacing (996 patients) and followed a median of 33.1 months. The primary endpoint was death from any cause or non-fatal stroke. Secondary endpoints included the composite of death, stroke, or hospitalization for heart failure; atrial fibrillation; heart-failure score; the pacemaker syndrome; and QoL.

Results: Death or non-fatal stroke rate was 21.5% in the dual chamber group and 23% in the ventricular-paced group (p = 0.48). In the dual chamber pacing group, the risk of atrial fibrillation was lower (HR 0.79; 95% CI 0.66 to 0.94; p = 0.008), and heart failure scores were better (p<0.001). The differences in the rates of hospitalization for heart failure and of death, stroke, or hospitalization for heart failure were not significant in unadjusted analyses but marginally significant in adjusted analyses. Dual chamber pacing resulted in a small increase in the QoL compared with ventricular pacing.

Conclusion: Dual chamber pacing does not improve mortality or stroke-free survival compared with ventricular pacing in sinus node dysfunction but does reduce the risk of atrial fibrillation, reduce signs and symptoms of heart failure, and improve the QoL.

Impact on management of elderly patients: Dual chamber pacing offers significant improvement as compared with ventricular pacing so should be the preferred mode of pacing in sinus node dysfunction unless there are contraindications.

SAFE PACE (Syncope And Falls in the Elderly – Pacing And Carotid sinus Evaluation)

Reference: Kenny RA, Richardson DA, Steen N, Bexton RS, Shaw FE, Bond J (2001) Carotid sinus syndrome: a modifiable risk factor for non-accidental falls in older adults (SAFE PACE). *Am J Cardiol* **38**:1491–6.

Study question: Does cardiac pacing reduce subsequent falls in older patients who present with non-accidental falls and have cardioinhibitory response to carotid sinus stimulation?

Short answer: Yes.

Study population: Patients aged >50 years presenting to A&E with non-accidental fall(s). Exclusion criteria included cognitive impairment (MMSE <23/30), blindness, contraindication to CSM, medical explanation for fall (e.g. epilepsy, stroke, alcohol excess), receiving medications known to cause hypersensitive response to CSM.

Method: Eligible participants invited for assessment including CSM. If CSM revealed cardioinhibitory carotid sinus hypersensitivity (CICSH), randomized into 2 groups; one which had pacemaker fitted, the other a control group.

Results: 1624 patients eligible for CSM: 34% had CSH (17% vasodepressor, 16% cardioinhibitory or mixed). 175 patients randomized into pacemaker versus control groups; falls reduced by two-thirds in pacemaker group (216 vs 669). Pacemaker group also had fewer syncopal episodes (28 vs 47) and fewer injurious events (61 vs 202).

Conclusion: Cardiac pacing significantly reduces subsequent falls in older patients who present with non-accidental falls and have CICSH.

Impact on management of elderly patients: Patients with non-accidental falls should have further cardiovascular assessment including CSM and insertion of pacemaker if found to have CICSH.

PASE (PAcemaker Selection in the Elderly trial)

Reference: Lamas GA, Orav EJ, Stambler BS, Ellenbogen KA, Sgarbossa EB, Huang SK, *et al.* (1998) Quality of life and clinical outcomes in elderly patients treated with ventricular pacing as compared with dual-chamber pacing. *N Engl J Med* **338**:1097–104.

Study question: Which pacing mode (ventricular or dual chamber pacing) improves QoL and reduces cardiovascular morbidity and mortality in the elderly?

Short answer: No difference between the 2 pacing modes except in sinus node dysfunction.

Study population: Patients aged >65 who were in sinus rhythm and required pacemaker for prevention or treatment of bradycardia (e.g. atrioventricular block or sinus-node dysfunction). Exclusion criteria included overt congestive heart failure at the time of implantation, permanent atrial fibrillation, serious non-cardiac illness and inadequate atrial-capture/sensing thresholds.

Method: All 407 participants had dual chamber, rate-adaptive pacemaker implanted. Randomized to 2 groups, one to have the pacemaker programmed to ventricular pacing, the other to dual chamber pacing. Participants' health status was assessed using Medical Outcomes Study Short-Form General Health Survey before randomization, then on 4 occasions up to the end of the trial 2 years later.

Results: Pacemaker implantation resulted in significant improvement in health-related QoL in both groups, with no difference between the groups. 26% of ventricular pacing participants were reprogrammed to dual chamber pacing after experiencing pacemaker syndrome. No significant differences between the 2 groups in rates of death, stroke or hospitalization for heart failure. Subgroup analysis revealed a favourable response of participants with sinus node dysfunction to dual chamber pacing.

Conclusion: Pacemaker implantation improves health-related QoL. Patients with sinus node dysfunction have greater QoL benefits from dual chamber pacing.

Impact on management of elderly patients: All patients found to have symptomatic atrioventricular block or sinus node dysfunction should be referred for pacemaker insertion.

Trials in cardiovascular risk modification

HYVET (Hypertension in the Very Elderly Trial)

Reference: Beckett NS, Peters R, Fletcher AE, Staessen JA, Liu L, Dumitrascu D, *et al.*; HYVET Study Group. (2008) Treatment of hypertension in patients 80 years of age or older. *N Engl J Med* **358**:1887–98.

Study question: Does treating hypertension in patients over 80 reduce their risk of stroke?

Short answer: Yes.

Method: Participants randomized into 2 groups – active treatment and placebo. Active treatment group received indapamide 1.5mg od (sustained release). If target BP of <150/<80 mmHg not reached, perindopril 2 mg od was added, increasing to perindopril 4 mg od if necessary. Participants followed up for mean 2.1 years. Primary endpoint was stroke. Secondary endpoints included death from any cause, cardiovascular or cardiac death.

Results: 3845 patients randomized (1933 active treatment, 1912 placebo). Active treatment resulted in 48.0% of patients reaching target BP, compared with 19.9% of placebo group (p <0.001). The active treatment group had fewer strokes (51 vs 69 per 1000 patient-years, p = 0.06) and fewer deaths from stroke (27 vs 42 per 1000 patient-years, p = 0.046). The active treatment group also had a lower rate of death from any cause (196 vs 235 per 1000 patient-years, p = 0.02) and lower heart failure event rate (22 vs 57 per 100 patient-years, p<0.001).

Conclusion: Antihypertensive treatment (indapamide ± perindopril) significantly reduces the risk of death from stroke and death from any cause in elderly patients.

Impact on management of elderly patients: Treating elderly hypertensive patients lowers their risk of death.

Syst-China (Systolic Hypertension in China trial)

Reference: Wang J, Staessen JA, Gong L, Liu L (2000) Chinese trial on isolated systolic hypertension in the elderly. Systolic Hypertension in China (Syst-China) Collaborative Group. *Arch Intern Med* **160**:211–20.

Study question: Does antihypertensive drug treatment reduce the incidence of fatal and nonfatal stroke in older Chinese patients with isolated systolic hypertension?

Short answer: Yes.

Study population: Chinese patients aged ≥60 with isolated systolic hypertension (BP 160–219/<95 mmHg). Exclusion criteria included severe concomitant cardiovascular or non-cardiovascular disease and renal failure (creatinine >180 μmol/l).

Results: Median follow-up was 3 years. Active treatment reduced the incidence of total mortality (HR 0.62; p <0.01), fatal and non-fatal stroke (HR 0.66; p <0.05), and all cardiovascular endpoints (HR 0.67; p<0.01).

Conclusion: In elderly Chinese patients with isolated systolic hypertension, stepwise antihypertensive treatment improves prognosis.

Impact on management of elderly patients: Elderly patients with isolated systolic hypertension should be treated with antihypertensive treatment to reduce cardiovascular events.

STOP-2 (Swedish Trial in Old Patients with Hypertension-2)

Reference: Hansson L, Lindholm LH, Ekbom T, Dahlöf B, Lanke J, Scherstén B, *et al.* (1999) Randomised trial of old and new antihypertensive drugs in elderly patients: cardiovascular mortality and morbidity the Swedish Trial in Old Patients with Hypertension-2 study. *Lancet* **354**:1751–6.

Study question: Are newer antihypertensive agents (ACE inhibitors, calcium antagonists) as efficacious as older agents (β-blockers, diuretics) in reducing cardiovascular mortality and morbidity in the elderly?

Short answer: Yes.

Study population: Hypertensive patients (BP ≥180 mmHg systolic or ≥105 mmHg diastolic or both) aged 70–84 years.

Method: Participants randomized into 3 treatment groups: group 1, β-blockers, diuretics, or both (atenolol 50 mg, metoprolol 100 mg, pindolol 5 mg or fixed-ratio hydrochlorothiazide 25 mg plus amiloride 2.5 mg); group 2, ACE inhibitors (enalapril 10 mg, lisinopril 10 mg); and group 3, calcium antagonists (felodipine 2.5 mg, isradipine 2.5 mg). BP recorded at start of trial and twice per year for the following 4 years. Endpoints (stroke, MI, cardiovascular mortality) assessed by independent committee.

Results: 6614 patients randomized: 2213 group 1, 2205 group 2, 2196 group 3. BP lowered by similar amount in each group (34.5–34.8/16.2–17.5 mmHg) and similar efficacy in prevention of cardiovascular mortality and major morbidity.

Conclusion: Older and newer agents are equally useful at lowering BP in elderly population.

Impact on management of elderly patients: Treating high BP in elderly patients lowers cardiovascular mortality, no matter which agent is used.

Syst-Eur (Systolic Hypertension in Europe trial)

Reference: Staessen JA, Fagard R, Thijs L, Celis H, Arabidze GG, Birkenhäger WH, *et al.* (1997) Randomised double-blind comparison of placebo and active treatment for older patients with isolated systolic hypertension. The Systolic Hypertension in Europe (Syst-Eur) Trial Investigators. *Lancet* **350**:757–64.

Study question: Does treating isolated systolic hypertension with nitrendipine ± enalapril ± hydrochlorothiazide reduce cardiovascular mortality and morbidity in the elderly?

Short answer: Yes.

Study population: European patients aged >60 years with isolated systolic hypertension (BP ≥160–219 mmHg systolic, diastolic <95 mmHg).

Method: Randomized into 2 groups: active treatment and placebo. Active treatment comprised nitrendipine combined with or replaced by enalapril or hydrochlorothiazide, or both, aiming to reduce systolic BP to <150 mmHg. Patients followed up for median 2 years. Endpoints were stroke, death, MI, congestive heart failure, renal insufficiency, and aortic aneurysm.

Results: 4695 patients randomized (2398 active treatment, 2297 placebo). Active treatment reduced the occurrence of all strokes by 42% (7.9 vs 13.7 strokes per 1000 patient-years) and deaths from cardiovascular causes (9.8 vs 13.5 deaths per 1000 patient-years).

Conclusion: Treatment of elderly patients with nitrendipine, enalapril, and hydrochlorothiazide reduced the risk of stroke and other cardiovascular complications.

Impact on management of elderly patients: Treating high systolic BP in elderly patients lowers cardiovascular mortality.

STONE (Shanghai Trial Of Nifedipine in the Elderly)

Reference: Gong L, Zhang W, Zhu Y, Zhu J, Kong D, Pagé V, et al. (1996) Shanghai Trial of Nifedipine in the Elderly (STONE). *J Hypertens* **14**:1237–45.

Study question: Does nifedipine reduce mortality and morbidity in elderly patients with hypertension?

Short answer: Yes.

Study population: Chinese patients aged 60–79 (mean 66) years with BP ≥160 mmHg systolic or ≥96 mmHg diastolic. Exclusion criteria were severe hypertension (systolic ≥220 mmHg or diastolic ≥125 mmHg), secondary hypertension, severe arrhythmia, stroke, angina, congestive heart failure, asthma, diabetes, or other significant disease.

Method: Participants allocated alternately into 2 groups: active treatment and placebo. Active treatment group treated with nifedipine 10 mg bd, titrating up to 60 mg/day until BP target of 140–159/<90 mmHg achieved. Additional treatment added (captopril 20–50 mg/day or dihydrochloro-thiazide 25 mg/day or both) if necessary to achieve target. Placebo group given matching tablets. Follow-up for 36 months. Outcome measures included stroke, CHF, MI, sudden death, and hospitalization.

Results: 1632 participants (817 nifedipine and 815 placebo). Incidence of cardiovascular events significantly lower in nifedipine group (32 vs 66, p = 0.0001), incidence of stroke and (24 vs 49 p = 0.0001) and severe arrhythmia (2 vs 10 p = 0.003) also significantly reduced. No significant reduction in cardiovascular deaths. The results should be interpreted with caution due to the trial design (single blind, sequential assignment) and most patients were <70 years.

Conclusion: Nifedipine ± captopril ± dihydrochlorothiazide reduces the incidence of severe clinical outcomes in hypertensive Chinese patients.

Impact on management of elderly patients: Treating older hypertensive patients with nifedipine lowers cardiovascular morbidity.

MRC trial of treating hypertension in older adults

Reference: Anon (1992) Medical Research Council trial of treatment of hypertension in older adults: principal results. MRC Working Party. *BMJ* **304**:405–12.

Study question: Does treatment with diuretic or B-blocker in hypertensive older adults reduces risk of stroke, coronary heart disease, and death?

Short answer: Yes.

Study population: 4396 patients aged 65–74 years with mean systolic blood pressure 160–209 mmHg and mean diastolic blood pressure <115 mmHg not taking antihypertensive therapy and recruited from general practices.

Method: Placebo-controlled, single-blind trial. Patients were randomized to a diuretic (hydrochlorothiazide 25 mg or 50 mg plus amiloride 2.5 mg or 5 mg daily), a B-blocker (atenolol 50 mg daily) or placebo. The main outcome measures were stroke, coronary events, and death from all causes.

Results: Both treatments reduced BP below the level in the placebo group. Compared with the placebo group, actively treated subjects (diuretic and B-blocker groups combined) had a 25% (95% CI 3% to 42%) reduction in stroke ($p = 0.04$), 19% (−2% to 36%) reduction in coronary events ($p = 0.08$), and 17% (2% to 29%) reduction in all cardiovascular events ($p = 0.03$). After adjusting for baseline characteristics the diuretic group had significantly reduced risks of stroke (31% (3% to 51%; $p = 0.04$), coronary events (44%; 21% to 60%; $p = 0.0009$), and all cardiovascular events (35%; 17% to 49%; $p = 0.0005$) compared with the placebo group. The B-blocker group showed no significant reductions in these endpoints.

Conclusion: Hydrochlorothiazide and amiloride reduce the risk of stroke, coronary events, and all cardiovascular events in older hypertensive adults.

Impact on management of elderly patients: Treating hypertension in the elderly with diuretic reduces vascular mortality and morbidity.

STOP-Hypertension (Swedish Trial in Old Patients with Hypertension)

Reference: Dahlöf B, Lindholm LH, Hansson L, Scherstén B, Ekbom T, Wester PO (1991) Morbidity and mortality in the Swedish Trial in old patients with hypertension (STOP-Hypertension). *Lancet* **338**:1281–5.

Study question: Does treatment of hypertension in the elderly reduce mortality and morbidity?

Short answer: Yes.

Study population: 1627 Swedish men and women aged 70–84 years recruited from health centres in Sweden, with systolic pressure between 180 and 230 mm Hg with a diastolic pressure of at least 90 mmHg, or a diastolic pressure between 105 and 120 mmHg irrespective of the systolic pressure.

Method: Randomized, double-blind study to compare the effects of active antihypertensive therapy (three B-blockers and one diuretic) and placebo on the frequency of fatal and non-fatal stroke, MI, and other cardiovascular death. The total duration of the study was 65 months and the average time in the study was 25 months. 812 patients were randomly allocated active treatment and 815 placebo.

Results: The mean difference in blood pressure between the active treatment and placebo groups at the last follow-up before an endpoint, death, or study termination was 19.5/8.1 mmHg. Compared with placebo, active treatment significantly reduced the number of primary endpoints (94 vs 58; p = 0.0031) and stroke morbidity and mortality (53 vs 29; p = 0.0081). There was a significantly reduced number of deaths in the active treatment group (63 vs 36; p = 0.0079). The benefits of treatment were discernible up to age 84 years.

Conclusion: Antihypertensive treatment in patients aged 70–84 years confers reduces cardiovascular morbidity and mortality and total mortality.

Impact on management of elderly patients: Treating hypertension in the elderly up to age 84 years reduces cardiovascular mortality and morbidity.

SHEP (Systolic Hypertension in the Elderly Program)

Reference: Anon (1991) Prevention of stroke by antihypertensive drug treatment in older persons with isolated systolic hypertension, SHEP Cooperative research group. *JAMA* **265**:3255–64.

Study question: Does treating isolated systolic hypertension reduce the risk of stroke?

Short answer: Yes.

Study population: Participants with systolic BP >160 mmHg and diastolic BP <90 mmHg aged ≥60 years. Exclusion criteria included major cardiovascular disease, cancer, established renal dysfunction, and alcoholic liver disease.

Method: Participants randomized into 2 groups: active treatment and placebo. Target BP was systolic <160 mmHg if initial reading was >180 mmHg or a reduction by 200 mmHg if initial systolic pressure was 160–179 mmHg. Active treatment comprised chlorthalidone 12.5 mg od, increased to 25 mg od if target BP not reached. Additional treatments to meet target BP were atenolol 25 mg od or reserpine 0.5 mg od (if atenolol contraindicated), increasing to 50 mg if necessary. Follow-up for 5 years. Primary outcome measure was stroke. Secondary outcome measures included cardiac death, MI, LVF, TIA, and renal dysfunction.

Results: 4736 patients randomized (2365 active treatment, 2371 placebo). Active treatment group had significantly fewer strokes (103 vs 159, relative risk 0.63). Absolute reduction in 5-year risk of stroke was 30 events per 1000 participants and total stroke incidence reduced by 36% in active treatment group (p = 0.0003). Active treatment group also had fewer episodes of MI (50 vs 74, relative risk 0.67), TIA (62 vs 82, relative risk 0.75), and LVF (48 vs 102, relative risk 0.46).

Conclusion: Treatment of isolated systolic hypertension in patients >60 years significantly reduces the risk of stroke and incidence of major cardiac and cardiovascular events.

Impact on management of elderly patients: Treating high systolic BP in elderly patients lowers incidence of stroke and cardiovascular events.

TONE (Trial Of Nonpharmacologic interventions in the Elderly)

Reference: Whelton PK, Appel LJ, Espeland MA, Applegate WB, Ettinger WH Jr, Kostis JB, *et al*. (1998) Sodium reduction and weight loss in the treatment of hypertension in older persons; A randomized controlled trial of nonpharmacologic interventions in the elderly (TONE). *JAMA* **279**:839–46.

Study question: Are weight loss and reduced sodium intake effective treatment options in older hypertensive patients?

Short answer: Yes.

Study population: 975 patients aged 60–80 years with BP <145 mmHg systolic and <85 mmHg diastolic on 1 antihypertensive or 1 combination antihypertensive agent. Exclusion criteria included recent MI/stroke, CHF, insulin-dependent diabetes mellitus, recent involuntary or unexplained weight loss.

Method: Participants divided into 2 groups: obese and non-obese. Subgroups were sodium reduction (144 obese, 196 non-obese), weight loss (147 obese only), sodium reduction and weight loss (147, obese only) and usual care (147 obese, 194 non-obese). Antihypertensive therapy was withdrawn at 3 months. Outcome measures: diagnosis of high BP at 1 or more follow-up visits, treatment with antihypertensive medication, or a cardiovascular event during follow-up (median 29 months).

Results: The combined outcome measure was reduced in reduced sodium intake groups (HR 0.69; p<0.001). Relative to usual care, HRs among the obese participants were 0.60 (p<0.001) for reduced sodium intake alone, 0.64 (p = 0.002) for weight loss alone, and 0.47 (p<0.001) for reduced sodium intake and weight loss combined. The frequency of cardiovascular events was similar in each of the 6 treatment groups. The study was limited as most of the patients were <70 years and had mild hypertension.

Conclusion: Sodium restriction and weight loss in obese subjects are effective and acceptable non-pharmacological approaches to control hypertension in the elderly treated with anti-hypertensive medication.

Impact on management of elderly patients: Non-pharmacological approach to control hypertension should be considered as an alternative or an adjunct to medication in elderly patients with mild hypertension.

PROSPER (Pravastatin in the elderly at risk of vascular disease)

Reference: Shepherd J, Blauw GJ, Murphy MB, Bollen EL, Buckley BM, Cobbe SM, *et al*; PROSPER study group. PROspective Study of Pravastatin in the Elderly at Risk (2002). Pravastatin in elderly individuals at risk of vascular disease (PROSPER): a randomised controlled trial. *Lancet* **360**:1623–30.

Study question: Does pravastatin reduce the risk of adverse cardiovascular events and cognitive decline in an elderly population with vascular risk factors?

Short answer: Yes, if the aim is to reduce coronary events.

Study population: 5804 patients aged 70–82 years with history of coronary artery disease, cerebrovascular disease or peripheral vascular disease, or risk factors for vascular disease (smoking, hypertension, diabetes). Baseline cholesterol of 4.0–9.0 mmol/l.

Method: Participants randomized into 2 groups: pravastatin (2891) and placebo (2913). Follow-up for 3 years; assessments including lipid profile, ECG, MMSE. Primary endpoints cardiac death, non-fatal MI, stroke.

Results: Pravastatin group had lower incidence (19% relative reduction) of coronary heart disease death or non-fatal MI (292 vs 356) but no significant reduction in stroke incidence (135 vs 131). Cognitive function declined at the same rate in both groups.

Conclusion: Pravastatin reduces the risk of coronary disease in patients with vascular disease or vascular risk factors. No reduction in stroke risk in this trial but short follow-up.

Impact on management of elderly patients: Statins should be considered for primary and secondary prevention of cardiovascular disease.

HOPE (Heart Outcomes Prevention Evaluation study)

Reference: Yusuf S, Sleight P, Pogue J, Bosch J, Davies R, Dagenais G (2000) Effects of an angiotensin-converting-enzyme inhibitor, ramipril, on cardiovascular events in high risk patients, Hope Investigators, *N Engl J Med* **342**:145–53.

Study question: Does ramipril reduce the risk of cardiovascular events in a high-risk population that does not have heart failure?

Short answer: Yes.

Study population: 9297 patients aged ≥55 years who had a history of coronary artery disease, stroke, peripheral vascular disease, or diabetes plus ≥1 other risk factor for cardiovascular disease (smoking, hypertension, ↑ total cholesterol, ↓ HDL, microalbuminuria). Exclusion criteria included known heart failure or ejection fraction <40%, current ACE inhibitor use, uncontrolled hypertension, or recent MI/stroke.

Method: Participants randomized into 3 groups: ramipril 10 mg od (4645 patients), placebo (4652) and ramipril 2.5 mg od (244). Planned follow-up for 6 years but study stopped early due to beneficial effects shown. Primary outcome measure was composite of death from cardiovascular causes, MI, and stroke.

Results: 5128 participants (55%) aged >65 years. Results consistent across subgroups. Ramipril 10 mg group had significantly fewer cardiovascular deaths, MIs, and strokes (14% vs 17.8%). Also fewer participants in ramipril group underwent revascularization (742 vs 852) but there was no reduction in likelihood of hospitalization for unstable angina. Commonest reason for stopping ramipril was cough (7.3% vs 1.8% placebo).

Conclusion: Ramipril reduces the risk of cardiovascular death, stroke, and MI in patients with vascular disease or vascular risk factors, but without heart failure.

Impact on management of elderly patients: Consider ACE inhibitor therapy for elderly patients with cardiovascular risk factors, regardless of whether they have heart failure or not.

Trials in atrial fibrillation

AFFIRM (Atrial Fibrillation Follow-up Investigation of Rhythm Management study)

Reference: The Atrial Fibrillation Follow-up Investigation of Rhythm Management (AFFIRM) Investigators (2002) A comparison of rate control and rhythm control in patients with atrial fibrillation. The Atrial Fibrillation Follow-up Investigation of Rhythm Management (AFFIRM) study. *N Engl J Med* **347**:1825–33.

Study question: Is rhythm control superior to rate control in atrial fibrillation.

Short answer: No.

Study population: 4060 patients, mean, age, 69.7 ± 9.0 years, were enrolled in the study. 70.8% had a history of hypertension, and 38.2% had coronary artery disease.

Method: Randomized multicentre comparison of cardioversion and treatment with antiarrhythmic drugs to maintain sinus rhythm (rhythm control) versus the use of rate-controlling drugs (rate control).

Results: 5-year mortality was 23.8% in the rhythm control group and 21.3% in the rate-control group (HR 1.15; 95% CI 0.99 to 1.34; p = 0.08). More patients in the rhythm control group than in the rate control group were hospitalized, and there were more adverse drug effects in the rhythm control group. In both groups, the majority of strokes occurred after warfarin had been stopped or the INR was subtherapeutic.

Conclusion: A rhythm control strategy offers no survival advantage over rate control in atrial fibrillation. Anticoagulation should be continued in this group of high-risk patients.

Impact on management of elderly patients: Until better pharmacological agents become available rate control remains the first-line strategy for most elderly patients with atrial fibrillation.

BAFTA (Birmingham Atrial Fibrillation Treatment of the Aged Study)

Reference: Mant J, Hobbs FD, Fletcher K, Roalfe A, Fitzmaurice D, Lip GY, Murray E; BAFTA investigators; Midland Research Practices Network (MidReC) (2007) Warfarin versus aspirin for stroke prevention in an elderly community population with atrial fibrillation (the Birmingham Atrial Fibrillation Treatment of the Aged Study, BAFTA): a randomised controlled trial. *Lancet* **370**:493–503.

Study question: Does warfarin reduced risk of major stroke, arterial embolism, or other intracranial haemorrhage compared with aspirin in elderly patients with atrial fibrillation?

Short answer: Yes.

Study population: 973 patients aged 75 years or over (mean age 81.5 ± 4.2 years) with atrial fibrillation were recruited from primary care.

Method: Patients were randomly assigned to warfarin (target INR 2–3) or aspirin (75 mg per day). Follow-up was for a mean of 2.7 years (SD 1.2). The primary endpoint was fatal or disabling stroke (ischaemic or haemorrhagic), intracranial haemorrhage, or clinically significant arterial embolism. Analysis was by intention to treat.

Results: There were 24 primary events (21 strokes, two other intracranial haemorrhages, and one systemic embolus) in people assigned to warfarin and 48 primary events (44 strokes, one other intracranial haemorrhage, and three systemic emboli) in people assigned to aspirin (yearly risk 1.8% vs 3.8%, relative risk 0.48; 95% CI 0.28 to 0.80; p = 0.003; absolute yearly risk reduction 2%; 95% CI 0.7 to 3.2). Yearly risk of extracranial haemorrhage was 1.4% (warfarin) versus 1.6% (aspirin) (relative risk 0.87; 0.43 to 1.73; absolute risk reduction 0.2%; –0.7 to 1.2).

Conclusion: Warfarin is 65% more effective than aspirin in reducing risk of stroke in elderly patients with atrial fibrillation with no significant difference in bleeding risk.

Impact on management of elderly patients: Anticoagulation therapy should be prescribed for people aged over 75 who have atrial fibrillation unless there are contraindications or the patient decides that the benefits are not worth the inconvenience.

Re-LY (Dabigatran versus warfarin in patients with atrial fibrillation)

Reference: Connolly SJ, Ezekowitz MD, Yusuf S, Eikelboom J, Oldgren J, *et al.*; RE-LY Steering Committee and Investigators (2009) Dabigatran versus warfarin in patients with atrial fibrillation. *N Engl J Med* **361**:1139–51.

Study question: Is dabigatran, a new oral direct thrombin inhibitor as effective as warfarin in reducing risk of stroke in patients with atrial fibrillation?

Short answer: Yes.

Study population: 18 113 patients with atrial fibrillation and at risk of stroke.

Method: A non-inferiority trial in which patients were randomly assigned to receive, in a blinded fashion, fixed doses of dabigatran 110 mg or 150 mg twice daily or, in an unblinded fashion, adjusted-dose warfarin. The median duration of the follow-up period was 2.0 years. The primary outcome was stroke or systemic embolism.

Results: The primary outcome rate was 1.69% per year in the warfarin group compared with 1.53% per year in the group that received 110 mg of dabigatran (relative risk with dabigatran 0.91; 95% CI 0.74 to 1.11; p<0.001 for non-inferiority) and 1.11% per year in the group that received 150 mg of dabigatran (relative risk 0.66; 95% CI 0.53 to 0.82; p<0.001 for superiority). The rate of major bleeding was 3.36% per year in the warfarin group, compared with 2.71% per year in the group receiving 110 mg of dabigatran (p = 0.003) and 3.11% per year in the group receiving 150 mg of dabigatran (p = 0.31). The rate of haemorrhagic stroke was 0.38% per year in the warfarin group, compared with 0.12% per year with 110 mg (p<0.001) and 0.10% per year with 150 mg of dabigatran (p <0.001). The mortality rate was not significantly different (4.13% per year in the warfarin group, 3.75% per year with 110 mg of dabigatran (p = 0.13), and 3.64% per year with 150 mg of dabigatran (p = 0.051)).

Conclusion: In patients with atrial fibrillation, dabigatran 110 mg was associated with rates of stroke and systemic embolism similar to those associated with warfarin, and lower rates of major haemorrhage. Dabigatran 150 mg was associated with lower rates of stroke and systemic embolism and similar rates of major haemorrhage compared with warfarin.

Impact on management of elderly patients: Dabigatran may be a useful alternative to warfarin in elderly patients with atrial fibrillation but is not yet approved for widespread use.

SPORTIF V (Ximelagatran vs warfarin for stroke prevention in patients with non-valvular atrial fibrillation)

Reference: Albers GW, Diener HC, Frison L, Grind M, Nevinson M, Partridge S, et al.; SPORTIF Executive Steering Committee for the SPORTIF V Investigators (2005) Ximelagatran vs warfarin for stroke prevention in patients with nonvalvular atrial fibrillation. A randomized trial. *JAMA* **293**:690–8.

Study question: Is the oral direct thrombin inhibitor ximelagatran as effective as warfarin for prevention of stroke and systemic embolism in patients with atrial fibrillation?

Short answer: Yes but there are concerns regarding hepatotoxicity.

Study population: Multicentre trial conducted at 409 North American sites, involving 3922 patients with non-valvular atrial fibrillation and additional stroke risk factors. Mean age was 72 ± 9.1 years and 42% were over 75 years of age.

Method: Non-inferiority, double-blind, randomized trial in which patients were randomized to adjusted-dose warfarin (aiming for an INR of 2.0–3.0) or fixed-dose oral ximelagatran, 36 mg twice daily. The primary endpoint was all strokes (ischaemic or haemorrhagic) and systemic embolic events.

Results: The primary event rate with ximelagatran was 1.6% per year and with warfarin was 1.2% per year (absolute difference 0.45% per year; 95% CI −0.13% to 1.03% per year; p <0.001 for the predefined non-inferiority hypothesis). When all-cause mortality was included in addition to stroke and systemic embolic events, the rate difference was not significant. There was no difference between treatment groups in rates of major bleeding, but total bleeding (major and minor) was lower with ximelagatran (37% vs 47% per year; 95% CI for the difference −14% to −6.0% per year; p<0.001). Serum ALT levels rose to greater than 3 times the upper limit of normal in 6.0% treated with ximelagatran, usually within 6 months. The mean INR with warfarin (2.4 ± 0.8) was within target during 68% of the treatment period.

Conclusion: Fixed-dose oral ximelagatran without coagulation monitoring is as effective as well-controlled warfarin for prevention of thrombo-embolism in patients with atrial fibrillation, but the potential for hepatotoxicity requires further investigation.

Impact on management of elderly patients: Fixed-dose oral ximelagatran may prove useful as an alternative to warfarin if hepatotoxicity does not prove to be a major problem.

EAFT (European Atrial Fibrillation Trial)

Reference: Anon (1993) Secondary prevention in non-rheumatic atrial fibrillation after transient ischaemic attack or minor stroke. EAFT (European Atrial Fibrillation Trial) Study Group. *Lancet* **342**:1255–62.

Study question: Does anticoagulation with warfarin or aspirin reduce the risk of stroke in patients with non-rheumatic atrial fibrillation (NRAF) who have had a recent TIA or minor stroke?

Short answer: Yes.

Study population: 1007 patients with NRAF and a recent TIA or minor ischaemic stroke.

Method: 669 patients were randomized to open anticoagulation or double-blind treatment with either 300 mg aspirin or placebo (group 1). 338 patients with contraindications to anticoagulation were randomized to receive aspirin or placebo (group 2). Outcome measure was death from vascular disease, any stroke, MI, or systemic embolism.

Results: During mean follow-up of 2.3 years, the annual rate of outcome events was 8% in patients assigned to anticoagulants versus 17% in placebo-treated patients in group 1 (HR 0.53; 95% CI 0.36 to 0.79). The risk of stroke alone was reduced from 12% to 4% per year (HR 0.34; 95% CI 0.20 to 0.57). Among all patients assigned to aspirin (groups 1 and 2), the annual incidence of outcome events was 15%, against 19% in those on placebo (HR 0.83; 95% CI 0.65 to 1.05). Anticoagulation was significantly more effective than aspirin (HR 0.60; 95% CI 0.41 to 0.87). The incidence of major bleeding events was low, both on anticoagulation (2.8% per year) and on aspirin (0.9% per year).

Conclusion: Anticoagulation with warfarin is effective in reducing the risk of recurrent vascular events in NRAF patients with a recent TIA or minor ischaemic stroke. Aspirin is a safe, though less effective, alternative when anticoagulation is contraindicated. Warfarin prevents 90 vascular events per 1000 patients treated per year compared with 40 for aspirin.

Impact on management of elderly patients: Patients with NRAF who present with TIA or minor stroke should be anticoagulated with warfarin unless there are contraindications when aspirin 300mg is an alternative.

Cochrane database review of primary prevention of stroke in non-rheumatic atrial fibrillation

Reference: Aguilar MI, Hart R, Pearce LA (2007). Oral anticoagulants versus antiplatelet therapy for preventing stroke in patients with non-valvular atrial fibrillation and no history of stroke or transient ischemic attacks. *Cochrane Database Syst Rev* (**3**):CD006186.

Study question: What is the relative effect of long-term oral anticoagulant treatment compared with antiplatelet therapy on major vascular events in patients with non-valvular AF and no history of stroke or TIA?

Short answer: Oral anticoagulant therapy is superior to aspirin.

Study population: All randomized trials in which long-term (more than four weeks) adjusted-dose oral anticoagulant treatment was compared with antiplatelet therapy in patients with chronic non-valvular AF.

Method: Two review authors independently selected trials for inclusion, assessed quality and extracted data.

Results: Eight randomized trials, including 9598 patients, tested adjusted-dose warfarin versus aspirin (in dosages ranging from 75 to 325 mg/day) in AF patients without prior stroke or TIA. The mean overall follow up was 1.9 years/participant. Oral anticoagulants were associated with lower risk of all stroke (OR 0.68; 95% CI 0.54 to 0.85), ischemic stroke (OR 0.53; 95% CI 0.41 to 0.68) and systemic emboli (OR 0.48; 95% CI 0.25 to 0.90). All disabling or fatal strokes (OR 0.71; 95% CI 0.59 to 1.04) and MI (OR 0.69; 95% CI 0.47 to 1.01) were reduced but not significantly by oral anticoagulants. Vascular death (OR 0.93; 95% CI 0.75 to 1.15) and all-cause mortality (OR 0.99; 95% CI 0.83 to 1.18), were similar with these treatments. Intracranial haemorrhages (OR 1.98; 95% CI 1.20 to 3.28) were increased by oral anticoagulant therapy.

Conclusion: Adjusted-dose warfarin and related oral anticoagulants reduce stroke, disabling stroke, and other major vascular events for those with non-valvular AF by about a third when compared with antiplatelet therapy.

Impact on management of elderly patients: Patients with non-rheumatic atrial fibrillation at increased risk of stroke should be prescribed anticoagulation with warfarin unless contraindicated or patient decides that the benefits are not worth the inconvenience.

ATHENA (Effect of dronedarone on cardiovascular events in atrial fibrillation)

Reference: Hohnloser SH, Crijns HJ, van Eickels M, Gaudin C, Page RL, Torp-Pedersen C, Connolly SJ; ATHENA Investigators (2009) Effect of dronedarone on cardiovascular events in atrial fibrillation. *N Engl J Med* **360**:668–78.

Study question: Does dronedarone, a new multichannel blocking antiarrhythmic drug reduce cardiovascular events in patients with atrial fibrillation?

Short answer: Yes.

Study population: A multicentre trial in 4628 patients with persistent or paroxysmal atrial fibrillation and at least 1 additional risk factor (age overt 70 years; arterial hypertension; diabetes mellitus; previous stroke or systemic embolism; left atrial enlargement; or LVEF ≤40%).

Method: Patients were randomly assigned to receive dronedarone, 400 mg twice a day (2301), or placebo (2307) in double-blind fashion. The primary outcome was the first hospitalization due to cardiovascular events or death. Secondary outcomes were death from any cause, death from cardiovascular causes, and hospitalization due to cardiovascular events.

Results: The mean follow-up was 21 ± 5 months. The study drug was discontinued prematurely in 30.2% receiving dronedarone and 30.8% receiving placebo, mostly because of adverse events. The primary outcome occurred in 31.9% in the dronedarone group and in 39.4% in the placebo group, with an HR for dronedarone of 0.76 (95% CI 0.69 to 0.84; p <0.001). Total mortality was 5.0% in the dronedarone group and 6.0% in the placebo group (HR 0.84; 95% CI 0.66 to 1.08; p = 0.18). Cardiovascular deaths were 2.7% in the dronedarone group and 3.9% in the placebo group (HR 0.71; 95% CI 0.51 to 0.98; p = 0.03), largely due to a reduction in arrhythmia deaths. The dronedarone group had higher rates of bradycardia, QT-interval prolongation, nausea, diarrhoea, rash, and increased serum creatinine level but thyroid- and pulmonary-related adverse events were not significantly different between the two groups.

Conclusion: Dronedarone reduced the incidence of hospitalization due to cardiovascular events or death in patients with atrial fibrillation.

Impact on management of elderly patients: Dronedarone may be a viable, effective, and safer treatment option for patients with atrial fibrillation and is under review by NICE (guidance due June 2010). It should not be used in severe heart failure.

Chapter 12

The elderly cardiac patient undergoing non-cardiac surgery

Non-cardiac surgery

Cardiovascular events during and after non-cardiac surgery contribute significantly to mortality and morbidity in the elderly. One in 5 patients over 70 years of age undergoing non-cardiac surgery will experience one or more serious postoperative complications.

The primary risk factor is not age. The strongest predictors of postoperative adverse events are cardiac disease (heart failure and arrhythmia) and reduced functional capacity. Pulmonary and neurological conditions are also important. Some of these factors are potentially modifiable and comprehensive preoperative assessment may prevent adverse postoperative outcomes.

The role of the cardiologist or geriatrician is not to pronounce the patient 'fit for anaesthesia'. The anaesthetist is ultimately responsible for this decision. The aim of preoperative assessment is to:

• Evaluate and assess the perioperative cardiac risk and provide information to the patient, surgeon, and anaesthetist to facilitate decision making
• Determine if further cardiac investigation and or treatment are indicated
• Provide recommendations on reducing the patient's perioperative risk by optimizing cardiac, renal, pulmonary, and general medical status preoperatively
• Assess and intervene to modify the long-term risk of cardiovascular disease.

Available guidelines

Over the years a number of risk scoring systems and guidelines have been developed for cardiovascular evaluation prior to non-cardiac surgery. The currently most used ones are:

- The Joint American College of Cardiology/American Heart Association (ACC/AHA) guidelines.
- The European Society Cardiology guidelines.
- The American College of Physicians (ACP) guidelines.
- The Association of Anaesthetists of Great Britain and Ireland: *Preoperative assessment and patient preparation. The role of the anaesthetist.*
- The Association of Anaesthetists of Great Britain and Ireland: *Anaesthesia and peri-operative care of the elderly.*
- The American Society of Anesthesiologists (ASA) classification of physical status (Table 12.1). This has a low specificity. Up to 50% of elderly patients are classed as high risk (III or above) and most of these patients will not have complications.
- The Revised Cardiac Risk Index (Lee *et al.* 1999).

Table 12.1 American Society of Anethesiologists Classification (ASA) of physical status

Class I	Normal healthy patient
Class II	Mild systemic disease (e.g. diabetes, hypertension)
Class III	Severe systemic disease (e.g. prior myocardial infarction)
Class IV	Life-threatening systemic disorder (e.g. end-stage chronic obstructive pulmonary disease)
Class V	Moribund patient needing a life-saving operation
Class VI	Brain-dead patient whose organs are been removed for donor purposes

Most of the guidelines and risk scores focus on ischaemic heart disease but other cardiac conditions are also important. This chapter initially concentrates on ischaemic heart disease but will also discuss other cardiac conditions such as valve disease, pacemakers, and medication management in the perioperative period. As many elderly patients have multiple comorbidities that are likely to influence outcome we would recommend the use of the **Comprehensive Geriatric Assessment (CGA)** as employed by the **Proactive Care of Older People undergoing surgery (POPS) project** in evaluating elderly patients preoperatively. The cardiovascular risk assessment can be included as part of this assessment.

The **POPS** project was designed at St Thomas' Hospital in London and showed that preoperative **CGA** incorporating prediction of adverse outcomes combined with targeted interventions reduced postoperative complications (including delirium and pneumonia) and length of stay in elective orthopaedic patients aged 65 years and over (Harari *et al.* 2007). The team included a consultant geriatrician, nurse specialist, occupational therapist, physiotherapist, and social worker. The criteria set by POPS for considering patients for preoperative assessment are outlined in Table 12.2.

Table 12.2 The Proactive Care of Older People undergoing surgery (POPS) project criteria for considering patients for preoperative assessment

Patients aged 65+ awaiting surgery, with any of the following:

Cardiovascular: myocardial infarction in past 2 years, unstable angina, untreated heart failure, untreated blood pressure >160/90 mmHg

Poorly controlled diabetes

Previous stroke

On warfarin

Chronic lung disease (if thought to put patient at risk)

Poor nutrition (body mass index <20, weight loss >5 kg in last 6 months)

Memory problems, history of confusion or known dementia

Activities of daily living (ADLs): needing help with getting to toilet, bed to chair, standing, dressing, walking. Likely to need a complex discharge package

The components of a Comprehensive Geriatric Assessment (Ellis and Langhorne 2005) are shown in Table 12.3.

Table 12.3 Components of a Comprehensive Geriatric Assessment (CGA)

Components	Elements
Medical assessment	Problem list
	Co-morbid conditions and disease severity
	Medication review
	Nutritional status
Assessment of functioning	Basic activities of daily living
	Instrumental activities of daily living
	Activity/exercise status
	Gait and balance
Psychological assessment	Mental status (cognitive) testing
	Mood/depression testing
Social assessment	Informal support needs and assets
	Care resource eligibility/financial assessment
Environmental assessment	Home safety
	Transportation and tele-health

Establishing a cardiovascular risk profile

The three major parameters that determine the risk of cardiac morbidity and mortality for patients undergoing non-cardiac surgery are:

• The clinical characteristics of the patient
• The inherent cardiac risk of the planned surgical procedure
• The patient's functional capacity.

The 2007 ACC/AHA guidelines recommend five key steps to assess risk.

Step 1: Is there a clinical need for emergency non-cardiac surgery?

If emergency surgical intervention is required (e.g. ruptured abdominal aortic aneurysm, acute subdural hematoma with papilloedema) surgery should proceed as soon as possible after stabilization. Preoperative cardiac testing will not only delay potentially life-saving surgery but also yield results that cannot be immediately addressed.

Step 2: Are there active cardiac conditions?

Clinical predictors of high risk include:

• Acute coronary syndromes (ACS) in last 30 days
• Class III or IV angina (Table 12.4)
• Decompensated heart failure
• Significant arrhythmias (high-grade atrioventricular (AV) block, symptomatic ventricular tachycardia and supraventricular arrhythmias with poor rate control)
• Severe valve disease (aortic or mitral stenosis).

Table 12.4 Canadian Cardiovascular Society Angina Classification

Class 0	Asymptomatic
Class I	Angina with strenuous exertion
Class II	Angina with moderate exertion
Class III	Angina with mild exertion
Class IV	Angina at rest or on any exertion

If any of these are present, patients should have further evaluation and treatment prior to elective surgery (see below). The extent of the assessment depends on the individual patient and the procedure to be performed. Where possible elective surgery should be deferred for at least 1 month and preferably 6 months after acute myocardial infarction or troponin-positive ACS.

Step 3: Does the planned surgery have a low cardiac risk?

Surgical procedures with <1% risk for cardiac death and non-fatal myocardial infarction are considered to be low risk (Table 12.5). Other minimally invasive surgical procedures performed on an ambulatory basis fall within the low-risk category. For these low-risk procedures, patients do not require further cardiac evaluation or treatment prior to surgery.

Table 12.5 Estimated risk of cardiac complications of surgery

High-risk surgery (cardiac risk >5%)
Emergency surgery (especially over age 75 years)
Cardiac procedures
Aortic or other major vascular procedures
Peripheral arterial vascular procedures
Prolonged surgery anticipated (>2 hours)
Anticipated large fluid shift or blood loss, e.g. Whipple's procedure, major spinal surgery
Intermediate-risk surgery (cardiac risk 1–5%)
Orthopaedic surgery
Urological surgery
Uncomplicated abdominal or thoracic surgery
Uncomplicated head and neck surgery
Carotid endarterectomy
Prostate surgery
Low-risk surgery (cardiac risk <1%)
Endoscopy
Bronchoscopy
Hysteroscopy
Cystoscopy
Dermatological procedures (skin and subcutaneous tissue)
Breast biopsy and other breast surgery
Ophthalmological procedures (e.g. cataract extraction)

Step 4: Does the patient have good functional capacity without symptoms?

Functional status is a reliable predictor of both perioperative and long-term cardiac risk. Functional capacity is generally defined on the basis of metabolic equivalent (MET) levels (Fig. 12.1). In many patients this can be easily determined from the clinical history using two simple questions: (1) Can you walk four blocks without stopping because of limiting symptoms? (2) Can you climb two flights of stairs without stopping because of limiting symptoms? Such activities indicate a level of 4–5 METs, which is equivalent to the physiological stress of most non-cardiac surgical procedures requiring general anaesthesia. Patients with good functional capacity can proceed with their planned surgery without further assessment or treatment.

All patients for major surgery should have METs > 4

Duke Activity Index

1 MET

Can you take care of yourself?
Eat, dress, or use the toilet?
Walk indoors around the house?
Walk a block or two on level ground
at 2 to 3 mph or 3.2 to 4.8 km per h?

Do light work around the house like
4 METs dusting or washing dishes?

4 METs

Climb a flight of stairs or walk up a hill?
Walk on level ground at 4 mph or 6.4 km/h?
Run a short distance?

Do heavy work around the house like scrubbing
floors or lifting or moving heavy furniture?

Participate in moderate recreational activities
like golf, bowling, dancing, doubles tennis, or
throwing a baseball or football?

>10 METs

Participate in strenuous sports like swimming,
singles tennis, football, basketball, or skiing?

Fig. 12.1 Functional capacity. All patients for major surgery should have metabolic equivalents (METs) >4.

Step 5: Does the patient have clinical risk factors?

The clinical risk factors that predict increased cardiovascular mortality and morbidity with non-cardiac surgery are shown in Table 12.6.

Table 12.6 Clinical risk factors that predict risk of cardiac death and non-fatal myocardial infarction with non-cardiac surgery

Condition	Examples
History of ischaemic heart disease	Previous MI or ACS(>30days)
	Previous positive stress test
	Angina
	Previous PCI or CABG
	ECG evidence of previous MI
History of compensated congestive heart failure	History of heart failure
	Previous pulmonary oedema
	CXR evidence of heart failure
History of cerebrovascular disease	Previous TIA or stroke
Diabetes mellitus	
Renal impairment	Creatinine >180 Mmol/l

MI, myocardial infarction; ACS, acute coronary syndromes; PCI, percutaneous coronary intervention; CABG, coronary artery bypass graft; CXR, chest radiograph; ECG, electrocardiogram; TIA, transient ischaemic attack.

If none of these clinical risk factors are present the patient should proceed with the planned non-cardiac surgery without further preoperative cardiac assessment as the anticipated risk of a major adverse perioperative cardiac event complicating a non-cardiac surgical procedure would be approximately 0.5%.

If the patient has one or more clinical risk factor, more extensive perioperative cardiac assessment may be warranted. In most patients this will involve using β-blockers to reduce excessive myocardial oxygen demand (see p.268). Non-invasive cardiac imaging with a view to revascularization is no longer routinely recommended especially in the elderly unless the results are likely to change subsequent management.

β-blockers to reduce cardiovascular risk

The evidence for use of β-blockers to reduce cardiovascular risk in non-cardiac surgery is still debated. Perioperative β-blocker therapy must be tailored to the individual patient aiming for a resting heart rate <65 beats/min. The potential hazards of β-blocker therapy are emphasized by the recently published results of the Peri-operative Ischemic Evaluation (POISE) trial. This trial excluded patients already on a β-blocker and patients whose physician planned to start a β-blocker, so must be interpreted in this light. Careful preoperative titration and postoperative clinical assessment is essential to avoid clinically significant hypotension and bradycardia, which were associated with increased 30-day perioperative mortality. An update on perioperative β-blocker therapy has recently been published by the ACC/AHA (2009).

Our current recommendations for β-blockers include:

• Patients receiving β-blockers to treat angina, heart failure, symptomatic arrhythmias, or hypertension should continue treatment. β-blockers should be administered on the day of surgery and continued with the least possible interruption throughout the perioperative period
• Patients with known ischaemic heart disease undergoing intermediate or high risk surgery
• Patients undergoing vascular surgery with evidence on history or non-invasive testing of ischaemic heart disease.

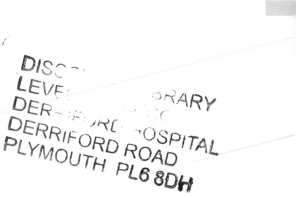

Coronary revascularization to reduce cardiovascular risk

As indicated above, non-invasive testing may be considered if the test results have potential to change patient management but routine preoperative stress testing is not recommended.

It is important to weigh the potential consequences of positive study findings and the need for revascularization with the potential risks of proceeding with non-cardiac surgery. This is especially relevant in the elderly where non-cardiac surgery is often performed to improve quality rather than quantity of life and where the risks of revascularization procedures are generally higher than in younger patients.

It has been assumed that revascularization in patients with severe ischaemia on non-invasive tests reduces the risk of non-cardiac surgery. However, this has been challenged by the results of two recent randomized controlled trials. The Coronary Artery Revascularization Prophylaxis (CARP) trial and the Decrease–V pilot study have both shown no benefit to revascularization prior to vascular surgery in patients with multiple clinical risk factors and significant ischaemia on stress imaging. The studies were small and further data are needed to define the role of revascularization and β-blocker therapy in this high-risk group.

Preoperative stress testing should be considered in the following groups if the results would change patient management in terms of revascularization prior to non-cardiac surgery, offering a different and less stressful non-cardiac procedure or non-surgical treatment:

- Patients with Class III/IV angina undergoing intermediate- or high-risk surgery.
- Patients undergoing vascular surgical procedures, particularly aorto-iliac and peripheral vascular surgery with multiple clinical risk factors (>3) (Table 12.6). These patients often have associated coronary disease that is asymptomatic due to the limitations of their peripheral vascular disease.
- Patients with myocardial infarction or ACS in the last 30 days undergoing intermediate- or high-risk surgery who have not had revascularization.
- Patients undergoing intermediate- or high-risk surgery with clinical risk factors and unable to tolerate β-blocker therapy.

The choice of non-invasive stress testing will depend on patient factors and local availability and expertise (Table 12.7).

If a noninvasive stress test, with or without imaging, yields severely abnormal results, the patient is usually referred for coronary angiography to determine the extent and severity of coronary heart disease (CHD). However this should not be the routine and rather the results should prompt modification of pharmacological therapy, close perioperative surveillance, and postoperative follow-up.

If angiography is performed, the indications for subsequent coronary bypass surgery (CABG) or percutaneous coronary intervention (PCI) are the same as in patients with chronic angina. See Chapter 2, p. 26 and p. 36.

Coronary revascularization is beneficial in patients with left main CHD and patients with three-vessel disease and impaired left ventricular function, and in selected patients with two-vessel disease and stenosis of the proximal left anterior descending artery. Revascularization in these patients has a long-term survival benefit, but it delays their non-cardiac surgery.

A delay of at least 4–8 weeks after coronary artery bypass grafting is usual before a patient can proceed with non-cardiac surgery and this is likely to be even longer in the elderly. Some elderly patients never recover sufficiently to proceed with non-cardiac surgery.

After PCI with bare metal stenting, 30 days of aspirin and clopidogrel therapy is recommended. Clopidogrel should be discontinued at least 7 days before surgery to reduce the risk of bleeding but aspirin should be continued unless the bleeding risk from surgery is very high (e.g. central nervous system surgery and prostate surgery).

After PCI with a drug-eluting stent, dual antiplatelet therapy (DAT) with aspirin and clopidogrel is recommended for 1 year.

If PCI is clinically indicated before non-cardiac surgery that cannot be delayed for 1 year, bare metal stent implantation is recommended, unless the bleeding risk of the procedure is low enough to permit DAT to be continued without interruption.

Patients who have had previous revascularization procedures who are asymptomatic or clinically stable with mild symptoms can be managed using the five-step approach (Establishing a cardiovascular risk profile, p. 264). β-blocker therapy should be prescribed especially if they have poor functional capacity and are undergoing intermediate-risk or high-risk surgery. Aspirin should be continued unless the bleeding risk of surgery is high as the cardiac risk associated with interruption of aspirin usually exceeds the risk of major bleeding. If aspirin is interrupted it should be restarted as soon as possible after surgery.

Table 12.7 Further tests to assess cardiac risk

Test	Potential value of results
Resting echocardiogram and Doppler	Not a good predictor of ischaemic events
	Useful in patients with CCF or suspected valve disease
Exercise stress testing	Measure functional capacity which can be impaired by age, deconditioning, myocardial ischaemia, and decreased cardiac or pulmonary reserve
	Development of ischaemia at a low workload is significant
	Elderly patients often cannot complete the test so the results are inconclusive
Pharmacological stress testing with nuclear imaging	Use thallium contrast and a pharmacological stressor such as adenosine or dipyridamole. Endpoints are the size and number of perfusion defects: fixed defects are less important than reversible defects for short-term prognosis
	Good negative predictive value (>95%) but poor positive predictive value (4–20%)
	Limited data on prognostic value in the elderly
Pharmacological stress testing with echocardiography	Use dobutamine as stressor and echocardiography to identify wall-motion abnormalities
	Evidence of ischaemia at low doses of dobutamine usually indicates severe disease. Negative predictive value is >93% but positive predictive value for serious events is only 7–25%

CCF, congestive cardiac failure.

Valve disease

Severe aortic and mitral stenosis are recognized as high risk for non-cardiac surgery.

Aortic stenosis

- The diagnosis is usually made clinically and confirmed by echocardiography.
- A transvalvular gradient of 50 mmHg or more is usually considered severe.
- In severe and symptomatic aortic stenosis (AS) elective non-cardiac surgery should be postponed or cancelled and consideration given to aortic valve replacement before non-cardiac surgery.
- The risk of valve replacement surgery in the elderly (Chapter 3, p. 50) must be considered in this situation.
- Percutaneous valve replacement (TAVI) may be an option in some patients if they otherwise meet the criteria for this procedure (Chapter 3, p. 52).
- If surgery is for malignant disease or other life-threatening conditions, it may be reasonable to proceed accepting the higher risk of non-cardiac surgery in these patients.
- If patients with severe AS proceed with non-cardiac surgery; careful intraoperative and perioperative monitoring is essential and care needs to be taken to avoid intraoperative hypotension. These patients are best managed in an intensive care (ITU)/high dependency (HDU) unit.
- Cardiac output is fairly fixed and these patients are very sensitive to volume depletion, blood loss, vasodilation, and arrhythmias so spinal anaesthesia and vasodilators are best avoided.

Mitral stenosis

- The clinical diagnosis may be difficult (Chapter 3, p. 60) and echocardiography is advised if the diagnosis is suspected.
- A valve area <1 cm^2 or gradient >20 mmHg is considered severe.
- If pulmonary hypertension is present the risk of general anaesthesia is significantly increased.
- Elective non-cardiac surgery should be postponed or cancelled if possible and consideration given to valvuloplasty or valve replacement surgery if otherwise indicated (Chapter 3, p. 60). The risk of cardiac surgery must also be considered.
- If non-cardiac surgery does proceed, careful intraoperative and perioperative monitoring is essential. These patients are best managed in ITU/HDU.

Other valve lesions

- Aortic and mitral regurgitation are generally not a contraindication to surgery unless heart failure is uncontrolled or left ventricular function is severely impaired.
- Advice on anticoagulation is provided on p. 282.
- Careful attention to fluid balance and rate control are essential in the perioperative period.
- Patients with well-functioning prosthetic valves can proceed with non-cardiac surgery.

Antibiotic prophylaxis for patients with valve disease undergoing non-cardiac surgery

- This subject has recently been reviewed by the National Institute for Health and Clinical Excellence (NICE).
- Current recommendations are that routine preoperative antibiotic prophylaxis for patients at risk of endocarditis is no longer recommended per se unless there are other reasons for it.
- Careful attention to dental and skin hygiene is recommended.
- There is still controversy about the guidelines and some people would still recommend prophylaxis in very-high-risk groups (e.g. prosthetic valves with previous endocarditis).
- Other recent guidelines are available from the AHA (2007) and the British Society of Antimicrobial Chemotherapy (BSAC 2006).
- Advice on the antibiotics to use should be obtained from local microbiologists or the BSAC guidelines.

The patient with heart failure

- Patients with CCF undergoing non-cardiac surgery have almost double the complication rate of patients with CAD.
- Patients with controlled CCF have an increased risk in high- and intermediate-risk surgery (Table 12.5).
- Medical therapy should be optimized preoperatively (Chapter 5).
- Careful attention to fluid balance and haemodynamic monitoring is essential in the perioperative period. These patients are best managed in ITU/HDU with involvement of cardiologists/physicians.
- Older patients with preserved systolic function but hypertrophied noncompliant ventricles can experience significant intraoperative and postoperative difficulties associated with fluid shifts, aggressive fluid administration, and possibly myocardial ischaemia.

Arrhythmias

- Cardiac arrhythmias that increase cardiovascular risk include high-grade AV block, symptomatic ventricular tachycardia, and supraventricular arrhythmias with poor rate control.
- Patients with Mobitz type 2 or complete heart block require insertion of a permanent pacemaker prior to elective non-cardiac surgery. If this is not possible a temporary pacemaker should be inserted for the peri-operative period.
- Patients with other arrhythmias should be managed as described in Chapters 6 and 7 and surgery deferred until the arrhythmia is controlled.

Pacemakers and devices

- Pacemakers and intracardiac defibrillators are increasingly used in the elderly.
- They are not a contraindication to surgery but the underlying cardiac condition needs to be considered.
- Most pacemakers are implanted to correct bradycardia due to sinus node disease or AV block but new indications include neurocardiogenic syncope, hypertrophic cardiomyopathy, and biventricular pacing in CCF.
- There are no nationally or internationally agreed guidelines for the management of patients with these devices in the perioperative period.
- Preoperatively it is important to check the type of device, the programmed settings, indication for implantation, and the patient's underlying rhythm.
- Routine preoperative checks are unnecessary if the device has been checked in the past 6 months and the information is available.
- If in doubt it is best to assume the patient is pacemaker dependent.
- Complications are rare but it is important to be aware of them and monitor carefully (Box 12.1).
- Ways to avoid complications are listed in Box 12.2.

Box 12.1 Potential complications of pacemakers and intracardiac defibrillators during non-cardiac surgery

- Pacemaker inhibition from unrecognized electromagnetic interference (EMI), usually diathermy or electrocautery. Most pacemakers recognize this and switch to asynchronous fixed rate pacing.
- Ventricular tracking of the interference signal leading to high rate pacing in patients with dual chamber pacing.
- Electrical reset of the pacemaker to demand or fixed rate pacing which persists after the interference has ceased.
- Very rarely irreversible damage to the device due to heat injury at the point of contact of the electrode and myocardium.
- EMI may be incorrectly detected as ventricular tachycardia/ventricular fibrillation by an intracardiac defibrillator, resulting in delivery of an inappropriate shock.
- The pacing or defibrillation thresholds may be altered by drugs, hypoxia, ischaemia, metabolic disturbance, or electrolyte imbalance.
- Damage to the device if external defibrillation is required. To avoid this place paddles in anteroposterior position or at least 10–15 cm away from the device.

Box 12.2 Avoiding complications with pacemakers and intracardiac defibrillators during non-cardiac surgery

- Keep the use and power output of electro-cautery to a minimum and avoid in close proximity to the device.
- Reprogramme defibrillators to a monitoring only mode with disabling of antitachycardia pacing and shock therapy perioperatively. If a programming device is not available this can also be achieved by application of a magnet.
- Temporary reprogramming to asynchronous or triggered mode in pacemaker-dependent patients if electrocautery needs to be used close to the device.
- Disable the rate-adaptive device if present.
- Careful monitoring and ready availability of emergency temporary or external pacing and defibrillation are important. If possible have appropriate programming equipment and magnets available for use provided there is available expertise in their use.
- If concerned that interference has occurred ensure the device is checked as soon as possible postoperatively and also ensure the patient is monitored until this can be done.

Hypertension

- Hypertension is common in the elderly and is not a contraindication to surgery.
- Moderate hypertension is not an independent risk factor for peri-operative complications.
- Severe hypertension (>160/110 mmHg) should be controlled prior to elective surgery (see Chapter 9).
- Ensure medication is continued unless contraindicated in the perioperative period.

Medication management

Antiplatelet therapy (aspirin, dipyridamole, and clopidogrel):

- There is a lack of data on stopping antiplatelet therapy preoperatively for patients on single-agent therapy.
- In patients with known ischaemic heart disease or cerebrovascular disease, aspirin should be continued unless the risk of bleeding is high (e.g. central nervous system surgery and prostate surgery).
- The decision should balance the consequences of perioperative haemorrhage against the risk of perioperative vascular complications.
- If therapy is interrupted the drug must be stopped at least 7 days preoperatively as platelet function takes 7–9 days to recover after cessation.
- It is also important to ask about non-prescribed therapies such as garlic, ginseng, and ginkgo, which also inhibit platelet function.

Dual antiplatelet therapy

- DAT with aspirin and clopidogrel is prescribed after ACS and PCI (see Coronary revascularization to reduce cardiovascular risk, p. 270).
- The combination increases the bleeding risk and interruption of therapy is associated with increased cardiac risk.
- If surgery is deemed essential the decision about interruption of therapy needs careful consideration and should be made by consultation with cardiologists, anaesthetists, and surgeons and the patient (see Coronary revascularization to reduce cardiovascular risk, p. 270).

Anticoagulation with warfarin

The management of the patient on warfarin depends on the clinical indication for warfarin. For patients with venous thrombo-embolism surgery should be avoided in the first month after the event if possible.

For elective surgery

- Stop for 4 days before surgery.
- Allow the international normalized ratio (INR) to fall below 1.5.
- Give low molecular weight heparin (LMWH) until 24 hours preoperatively or intravenous unfractionated heparin until 6 hours preoperatively if continued anticoagulation essential (e.g. mechanical valve). In patients with atrial fibrillation not at high risk of embolic events (markers of high risk include CCF, previous stroke, hypertension, and diabetes) heparin is not necessary in the preoperative period.
- Restart LMWH heparin 12 hours postoperatively or intravenous heparin 6 hours postoperatively if full anticoagulation required and the surgeon is happy that bleeding risk is low. The advantage of intravenous heparin is that it can be stopped immediately if bleeding occurs as there is no antidote to LMWH.
- Restart warfarin when oral intake possible.
- Stop heparin when INR therapeutic.

For emergency surgery
- Seek specialist advice.
- Give vitamin K ± fresh frozen plasma until INR reaches 1.5.
- In most cases it is preferable to use low dose vitamin K (1–2 mg) as this will interfere less with re-anticoagulation postoperatively.

Other cardiovascular drugs
- Antihypertensive, antianginals, and antiarrhythmics should be continued perioperatively in most patients.
- Potassium-sparing diuretics should be omitted on the day of surgery.
- There is some concern that patients on angiotensin-converting enzyme (ACE) inhibitors have more pronounced hypotension at induction and some anaesthetists omit the dose on the morning of surgery, but there is no consensus on this.
- Recently there has been interest in a role for statin therapy in reducing cardiovascular risk perioperatively. Most of the data are retrospective and to date only one small randomized controlled trial has been conducted so there is not enough evidence to recommend routine use of statins for this indication at present. Statins should be continued in patients already prescribed them.

Some common and important perioperative issues in the elderly

- The most common cardiac complications associated with surgery in the elderly are *myocardial infarction and myocardial ischaemia*. Myocardial infarctions (usually non-ST segment elevation (NSTEMI)) are most common in the first 3 days after surgery and are often painless. They may present with dyspnoea, hypotension, CCF, arrhythmia, and altered mental status in the elderly. Routine postoperative ECGs or troponin tests are not necessary but close monitoring and a high index of suspicion are needed, especially in high- and intermediate-risk patients.
- Patients with *valve disease* are especially sensitive to volume load and depletion and rapid heart rates so require careful haemodynamic and fluid balance monitoring in the perioperative period. This should include central venous pressure (CVP) and Doppler cardiac output monitoring if available. These patients should be monitored on an HDU or ITU postoperatively until stable.
- *Cardiac arrhythmias* are also common in the peri- and postoperative period in the elderly. They are often secondary to other problems including hypotension, electrolyte disturbance, hypoxia, acid–base disturbance, ischaemia, infection, heart failure, pulmonary embolism, drug reactions, which should be searched for and treated. They are often transient and require no other specific treatment. Persistent arrhythmias should be treated as outlined in the Chapters 6 and 7.
- *Delirium* or acute confusion is common in elderly patients postoperatively. A careful assessment of the precipitating cause and appropriate treatment are essential. Consider infection, electrolyte imbalance, medication change (new drug or withdrawal of existing therapy), alcohol withdrawal, etc. Sedation may be required if a patient is at risk of harming themselves or others and cannot be managed safely with non-pharmacological measures alone or for essential investigations to be performed. It is best to use low doses of a single agent such as lorazepam (or haloperidol if distressing psychotic symptoms) (see British Geriatrics Society and Royal College of Physicians 2006).

Important points to remember

- The risks of non-cardiac surgery are increased in the elderly but age itself is not a contraindication to surgery.
- The aim of preoperative assessment is to define the risk, optimize treatment where possible and allow an informed decision.
- Routine revascularization prior to non-cardiac surgery is not recommended at present.
- Patients on DAT need careful consideration.

Guidelines, references, and recommended reading

American College of Physicians (1997) Guidelines for assessing and managing the perioperative risk from coronary artery disease associated with major noncardiac surgery. *Ann Intern Med* **127**:309–12.

Association of Anaesthetists of Great Britain and Ireland (2001, planned update 2010) Anaesthesia and peri-operative care of the elderly. London: Association of Anaesthetists of Great Britain and Ireland. Available from: www.aagbi.org.

Association of Anaesthetists of Great Britain and Ireland (2010) Preoperative assessment and patient preparation. The role of the anaesthetist. London: Association of Anaesthetists of Great Britain and Ireland. Available from: www.aagbi.org.

British Geriatrics Society and Royal College of Physicians (2006) Guidelines for the prevention, diagnosis and management of delirium in older people. Concise guidance for good practice series, No. 6. London: Royal College of Physicians.

Ellis G, Langhorne P (2005) Comprehensive geriatric assessment for older hospital patients. *Br Med Bull* **71**:45–9.

Fleischmann KE, Beckman JA, Buller CE, Calkins H, Fleisher LA, Freeman WK, *et al.* (2009). 2009 ACCF/AHA focused update on perioperative beta blockade: a report of the American College Of Cardiology Foundation/American Heart Association Task Force on Practice Guidelines. *J Am College Cardiol* **54**:2102–28. Available from: www.americanheart.org.

Fleisher LA, Beckman JA, Brown KA, Calkins H, Chaikof EL, Fleischmann KE, Fet al.; American College of Cardiology; American Heart Association Task Force on Practice Guidelines (writing Committee to Revise the 2002 Guidelines on Perioperative Cardiovascular Evaluation for Noncardiac Surgery); American Society of Echocardiography; American Society of Nuclear Cardiology; Heart Rhythm Society; Society of Cardiovascular Anesthesiologists; Society for Cardiovascular Angiography and Interventions; Society for Vascular Medicine and Biology; Society for Vascular Surgery (2007) ACC/AHA 2007 guidelines on perioperative cardiovascular evaluation and care for noncardiac surgery: a report of the American College of Cardiology/American Heart Association Task Force on Practice Guidelines. *Circulation* **116**:1971–96. Available from: www.americanheart.org.

Gould FK, Elliott TS, Foweraker J, Fulford M, Perry JD, Roberts GJ, *et al.*, Working Party of the British Society for Antimicrobial Chemotherapy (2006) Guidelines for the prevention of endocarditis: report of the Working Party of the British Society for Antimicrobial Chemotherapy. *J Antimicrob Chemother* **57**:1035–42.

Harari D, Hopper A, Dhesi J, Babic-Illman G, Lockwood L, Martin F (2007) Proactive Care of older people undergoing surgery (POPS): Designing, embedding, evaluating and funding a comprehensive assessment service for older elective surgical patients. *Age Ageing* **36**: 190–6.

Lee TH, Marcantonio ER, Mangione CM, Thomas EJ, Polanczyk CA, Cook EF, *et al.* (1999) Derivation and prospective validation of a simple index for prediction of cardiac risk of major noncardiac surgery. *Circulation* **100**:1043–9.

McFalls EO, Ward HB, Moritz TE, Goldman S, Krupski WC, Littooy F, *et al.* (2004) Coronary-artery revascularization before elective major vascular surgery. *N Engl J Med* **351**:2795–804.

National Institute for Health and Clinical Excellence (2003) Pre-operative tests: the use of routine preoperative tests for elective surgery. Clinical guideline 3. London: National Institute for Health and Clinical Excellence. Available from: www.nice.org.uk/CG3.

National Institute for Health and Clinical Excellence (2008) Prophylaxis against infective endocarditis: antimicrobial prophylaxis against infective endocarditis in adults and children undergoing interventional procedures. Clinical guideline 64. London: National Institute for Health and Clinical Excellence. Available from: www.nice.org.uk/CG064.

Poldermans D, Schouten O, Vidakovic R, Bax JJ, Thomson IR, Hoeks SE, *et al.*; DECREASE Study Group (2007) A clinical randomized trial to evaluate the safety of a noninvasive approach in high-risk patients undergoing major vascular surgery: the DECREASE-V Pilot Study. *J Am Coll Cardiol* **49**:1763–9.

Poldermans D, Bax JJ, Boersma E, De Hert S, Eeckhout E, Fowkes G, *et al.*; Task Force for Preoperative Cardiac Risk Assessment and Perioperative Cardiac Management in Non-cardiac Surgery, European Society of Cardiology; European Society of Anaesthesiology (2009) Guidelines for pre-operative cardiac risk assessment and perioperative cardiac management in non-cardiac surgery: the Task Force for Preoperative Cardiac Risk Assessment and Perioperative Cardiac Management in Non-cardiac Surgery of the European Society of Cardiology (ESC) and endorsed by the European Society of Anaesthesiology (ESA). *Eur Heart J* **30**:2769–812. Available from: www.escardio.org/guidelines.

POISE Study Group, Devereaux PJ, Yang H, Yusuf S, Guyatt G, Leslie K, Villar JC, *et al.* (2008) Effects of extended-release metoprolol succinate in patients undergoing non-cardiac surgery (POISE trial): a randomised controlled trial. *Lancet* **371**:1839–47.

Wilson W, Taubert KA, Gewitz M, Lockhart PB, Baddour LM, Levison M, *et al.*; American Heart Association Rheumatic Fever, Endocarditis, and Kawasaki Disease Committee; American Heart Association Council on Cardiovascular Disease in the Young; American Heart Association Council on Clinical Cardiology; American Heart Association Council on Cardiovascular Surgery and Anesthesia; Quality of Care and Outcomes Research Interdisciplinary Working Group (2007) Prevention of infective endocarditis. Guidelines from the American Heart Association. *Circulation* **116**: 1736–54.

Chapter 13

Medical treatment and approaching end of life

Introduction

One of the roles of the doctor or health care professional is to decide when the end of life is imminent/approaching. Good end of life care is an important component in the care of older people whatever the diagnosis and this especially important in cardiovascular disease as many patients are elderly and will die from their disease.

Traditionally cardiovascular physicians have focused on active treatment of the disease and have been reluctant to address end of life issues until the terminal phase of the illness. The end of life care strategy (DOH, 2008) emphasizes the need for more proactive and advance care planning to improve end of life care.

Unfortunately in cardiovascular disease it can be difficult to apply prognostic criteria to individual patients e.g. heart failure has a fairly unpredictable course, with relapses and remissions making prognostic advice more difficult than in cancer care. The complex and diverse needs of patients with advanced cardiovascular disease require the collaborative effort of different specialties and professional groups. Palliative care seeks to influence improvement in the quality of life of patients with incurable disease by advocating a holistic, problem-orientated approach, including symptom control.

The frameworks of care developed in supportive and palliative care (the Gold Standards Framework and the Liverpool Care Pathway) are also relevant to improving collaborative working.

The role of the cardiologist/physician is:

- Advance care planning: open communication between all involved in the patient's care to discuss treatment decisions and ongoing care
- Honest prognostication: it is recognised that accurate prognostication can be difficult, especially for non-cancer patients, but some indication of time left may be very helpful to those patients and relatives who wish to know. Doctors are known to be frequently over-optimistic in estimating prognosis
- Making appropriate decisions regarding when to move from active treatment to palliative care – involving the MDT
- Co-ordinating care across palliative and primary care – need to be aware of local service provision
- Answer "experts" questions from the patient
- Symptom control and seeking help and advice from other professionals where necessary
- Review of medical therapy to improve quality of life
- Review of device therapy – see Chapter 5
- Commissioning, coordinating and developing services to improve end of life experience of patients with cardiovascular disease.

Ethical and legal aspects of end of life care

Many complex ethical decisions arise in the management of elderly people with chronic diseases. It is best to approach these with the help of the multidisciplinary team and the full involvement of the patient.

Ethical issues

Beauchamp and Childress introduced the concept of Principlism as a means of objectively approaching and weighing up difficult decisions. Their four principles are: autonomy, justice, beneficence and non-malfeasance, and have become widely accepted by clinicians as a good starting point within which to frame ethical decision making.

Autonomy

Respecting patients' wishes and facilitating and encouraging their input into the medical decision making process. To respect a patient's autonomy it is essential to explain, not only what is wrong with that person, but the options and implications of any proposed investigation and treatment and the associated risks and benefits. The issue of informed consent and refusal lies at the heart of this principle.

Justice

This implies an impartial and fair approach to treatment and the distribution of resources. Human rights codes condemn any form of discrimination on the grounds of age, race, sex, religion and sexual orientation.

Beneficence (to do good) and non-maleficence (to do no harm)

The doctor should act to promote the welfare of the patient and to do good (beneficence). However an action taken to benefit the patient may entail risks so at the same time doctor has to consider the principle of non-malfeasance (to do no harm).

Legal issues

Ethical decisions must be made within the existing legal framework. The following areas of law are of particular relevance to the older population:
- Mental Capacity Act
- Consent
- Confidentiality.

Mental Capacity Act (2005)

The right of any patient deemed to have capacity to refuse medical treatment is enshrined in UK law. However until recently, decisions made on behalf of those lacking capacity had no statutory framework. The Mental Capacity Act (MCA) has created this. Capacity decisions are therefore now legal decisions and certain categories of people have a legal duty to have regard to the code of practice. These include professionals and anyone who is paid for the work they do in relation to people who lack capacity eg: doctors, nurses, social workers, care managers, paid carers. The assessment of capacity to participate in research is identical to that for medical treatment.

Summary of the MCA

1. The MCA establishes five statutory principles (the majority of which were already widely used as they are derived from case law)

- A person must be assumed to have capacity unless established that he lacks capacity
- All practicable steps must be taken to enable a person to make a decision
- People can make unwise decisions
- An act done or a decision made on behalf of a person who lacks capacity must be done in his best interests
- All actions taken must be the least restrictive of the person's rights and freedom of action.

2. Establishes legal test of capacity

Capacity is time- and decision- specific. Decisions about capacity should be unrelated to a person's age, appearance, condition or behaviour. Capacity can be assessed by a two-stage test (Figure 13.1):

I: Does the person have a disturbance of the mind or brain (temporary or permanent) ie: what is your reason to suspect they may lack capacity?

II: Does that disturbance mean they are unable to make the decision in question at the time it needs to be made (apply a four stage test to determine this—see Figure 13.1)?

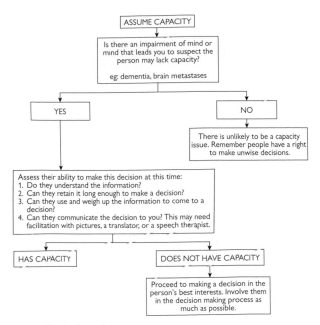

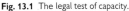

Fig. 13.1 The legal test of capacity.

3. Gives guidance in making 'best interests' decisions

If having applied the following tests of capacity a patient is deemed to lack capacity with regards to a specific decision, the choices made on their behalf should be in their best interests. The Act gives the following advice:

- Could the person regain capacity; can the decision wait?
- Encourage the person's participation to find out their views and consult others who know them; this would include anyone engaged in caring, friends or relatives and anyone appointed as attorney via an LPA (see below)
- If the person has no friends or family to consult, involve an IMCA (see below)
- Identify all relevant circumstances and avoid restricting the person's rights
- Avoid discrimination.

'Best interest' decisions can be extremely difficult; involve as many people as possible. In cases of extreme controversy or difficulty it may be necessary to seek legal advice and have the matter determined by judicial process. There are circumstances in which it may not be necessary to make a 'best interests' decision even for a person that lacks capacity. For example:

- Where an advance decision has been made by the person to refuse medical treatment
- The decision to involve a person who lacks capacity in a clinical trial may not be directly in their best interests.

4. Establishes new decision making mechanisms that have legal force

- Lasting Power of Attorney (LPA) (replaces enduring power of attorney). See Box 13.1
- Advance decisions to refuse treatment.
- Deprivation of Liberty Safeguards (added in 2007). See Box 13.2.

Box 13.1 Lasting Power of Attorney (LPA)

- For property and affairs (replaces old enduring power of attorney)
- And/or for welfare decisions including healthcare and place of residence.

Can be appointed whilst competent to make decisions in specified areas on behalf of the person when they lose capacity to do so themselves. Any decisions of the appointed person must still fulfill the best interests requirement.

At present, limited numbers of LPAs exist as the appointment procedure requires a solicitor, involves a complex form and is relatively expensive. Patients should be encouraged to appoint someone as their attorney via an LPA (if appropriate) during discussions around advance care planning (see p.298) whilst they still have capacity to do so.

Box 13.2 Deprivation of Liberty Safeguards (DOLS)

- Form an addition to the MCA
- Contain procedures for authorizing the deprivation of liberty in hospitals and care homes for patients that lack the capacity to consent to being there
- Developed in response to the Bournewood case and concerns the human rights (e.g.: Article 5 of the European Human Rights Act 1998: the right to liberty and security) of those who lack capacity may be jeopardized by the MCA
- The definitions within the safeguards are not clear and will be clarified over time as case law develops. e.g.: what exactly qualifies as 'deprivation'
- At present, it is practical to recognize that some patients who lack capacity will require a degree of restraint to ensure their safety and the safety of others
- The DOLS code of practice need only be used if that restraint is restrictive in its intensity or its cumulative effect over time
- Review under the DOLs code may conclude that the degree of restraint is necessary and proportionate – in which case it provides a clear process of review and appoints a representative to watch over the patient's interests in this area
- Every hospital and care facility should have DOLS protocol and staff trained in its application however the extent to which these safeguards are applied varies widely between institutions.

For example, a patient with severe dementia is mobile and repeatedly leaves the ward and wanders out onto the road outside the hospital. The doors to the ward are therefore locked, thus depriving him of his liberty. The DOLS code of practice should be used in this case to review whether this restraint is necessary and proportionate.

http://www.dh.gov.uk/en/SocialCare/Deliveringadultsocialcare/MentalCapacity/MentalCapacity
ActDeprivationofLibertySafeguards/index.htm

5. *Introduces the role of IMCA (see Box 13.3)*

Box 13.3 IMCA : Independent mental capacity advocate

- Appointed by healthcare professional to act in an advocacy role for any 'unbefriended' patient that lacks capacity (i.e.: no friends or family to assist best interest decisions)
- Legally required if decisions regarding serious medical treatment or change in accommodation are being made (see details below)
- Urgent treatment decisions which cannot wait for IMCA appointment can still be made by the medical team in the patient's best interests
- An IMCA is not required if the patient has made a valid and applicable advance decision to refuse treatment or has appointed someone as their decision maker via a lasting power of attorney (LPA)
- Usually provided by advocacy charities; each PCT has commissioned an IMCA service- local guidelines for referral will differ.

Decisions requiring IMCA involvement
- 1. Change in accommodation
  - Any decision to move a patient that lacks capacity to new accommodation provided by social services or NHS that is likely to last more than 8 weeks.
- 2. Hospital stay longer than 28 days
  - If there is a decision to be made as to whether to keep a patient in hospital for prolonged admission e.g.: inpatient rehabilitation
- 3. Serious medical treatment
  - Any treatment option that may have serious consequences or where the benefits and risks are finely balanced, or where there is a lack of consensus between clinical teams as to best treatment.

Consent

Patients who have capacity to make decisions must give consent for a medical treatment to be legal. For simple procedures this may be implied consent e.g., willingly offering their arm for a blood test. For more complex procedures and treatments a longer discussion with the patient is needed so that they can weigh up the risks and benefits before signing a consent form if necessary. Responsibility for seeking consent lies with the health-care professional undertaking an investigation or providing a treatment.

Common Law governs issues surrounding consent and is summarised at the end of the GMC booklet 'Consent: patients and doctors making decisions together'. As well as detailing the legal basis of consent, the GMC code establishes present best medical practice in this area.

For consent to be valid it must be:

Given by a person with capacity
See Figure 13.1.

Fully informed
It can be difficult to know how much information to give a patient in order to facilitate their decision-making, particularly in the elderly. GMC guidance states that:

- The amount of information about risk that you should share with patients will depend on the individual patient and what they want or need to know
- Discussions should include details of side effects, potential complications and failure of any intervention to achieve the desired outcome. Consequences of declining the treatment should also be discussed
- You must tell patients if an investigation or treatment might result in a serious adverse outcome even if the likelihood is very small. You should also tell patients about less serious side effects or complications if they occur frequently, and explain what the patient should do if they experience any of them
- Remember that patients are permitted to make decisions deemed 'unwise' by the medical team if they are fully informed and have capacity to do so.

Non-coerced
Patients may be put under pressure by carers, insurers, relatives or others, to accept a particular investigation or treatment. You should be particularly aware of this in the vulnerable elderly, especially those living in care facilities.

Confidentiality

Confidentiality is central to trust between doctors and patients. Again the GMC has published useful guidance in this area. Key points are:

- Doctors have a duty to keep any information learned in a professional capacity confidential
- Confidentiality is not an absolute duty and can be breached if required by law, justified in the public interest or if the patient consents
- Careful consideration must be given to breaking the confidence of a patient. Doctors must be able to justify these breaches
- Patients should be aware of what information has been divulged
- Information to be used in education, research or for public health interests should be anonymous where possible
- Seek the advice of your Caldicott Guardian if unsure about the use of patient information in any context.

End of life care for elderly patients with cardiovascular disease

The principles of end of life care in cardiovascular disease are identical to those in a patient suffering from cancer. However unlike most malignancies, cardiovascular disease runs an unpredictable course towards the end of life. For this reason planning in advance is even more critical. This is especially true in elderly patients developing cognitive impairment. The opportunity should be taken to establish their wishes before they lose capacity to make decisions. They may also choose to appoint a Lasting Power of Attorney (LPA). If a patient no longer has capacity and has not made any advance plans or appointed an LPA, decisions should be made in their best interests as described above.

Advance care planning (ACP)

ACP is an umbrella term used to refer to the personal, social and legal decisions that can be discussed and planned for in advance of their occurrence at the end of life. For example, writing a will or an advance decision, or discussing with your GP where your preferred place of care would be at the end of your life. This is a rapidly developing area in terms of documentation and legislation.

However the key is in the title, 'advanced'. These discussions and decisions should ideally be made well in advance of a crisis situation. As a result the burden of discussion should ideally fall to those healthcare professionals dealing with patients in non-acute settings e.g.: the GP surgery, the outpatient clinic, a specialist nurse. These discussions take time, and changes may need to be made to clinic schedules to facilitate them. A patient may choose to document their plans in an advance decision to refuse treatment (see Box 13.4).

Barriers to ACP

Fear of patient reaction

In reality it is often found that starting to talk about hopes and fears towards the end of life can be a relief for patients and their families. They have usually been thinking about it already. It is far preferable to initiate discussions in a controlled environment than when the patient is in extremis. Occasionally a patient may not wish to explore the topic further, but this in itself is useful to discover and be aware of.

Lack of training

Communication skills training increasingly forms a priority in undergraduate curricula, however ongoing revision is needed as part of continuing professional development. ACP is relevant in all areas of medicine from the emergency room to the mortuary and there is likely to be a working group in your hospital or PCT that can update you on what is happening in your area and direct you to good training. The following website has several excellent resources for advance care planning: www.endoflifecareforadults.nhs.uk.

Increased workload

ACP discussions cannot be rushed, and a culture-shift is needed to allocate adequate time to accommodate them within current service provision. Imaginative service development across primary and secondary care and often using the expertise of the palliative care services can revolutionise thi s area.

Oncology has led the way in this field but advance care planning is not just relevant to cancer care- any elderly person with a chronic life-limiting disease (COPD, heart failure, dementia, etc) should be given the chance to express and document their wishes for future care. ACP needs a 'champion' in each care setting to lobby for these changed priorities – perhaps it could be you?

Documentation

There is no standardized national document to facilitate ACP. As well as the advance decision document already mentioned, the 'Preferred Priorities of Care' document is a patient led document which has been well received: https://www.endoflifecareforadults.nhs.uk/wiki/files/F2110-Preferred_Priorities_for_Care_V2_Dec2007.pdf.

Box 13.4 Advance decisions to refuse treatment

- Have legal force since the MCA 2005
- Can only be made if over 18 and mentally competent
- Must specify the precise treatment that is being refused
- May be oral or in writing and may be altered orally
- BUT in order to refuse a lifesaving treatment, advance decision must be in writing and signed before a witness and the lifesaving treatment must be specified
- If an advance decision is valid and applicable, treatment cannot be given if the person loses capacity
- However advance decisions Can be overridden by Part IV of the Mental Health Act 2007, and any disputes that arise can be determined by the Court of Protection
- It is good practice for a patient to keep a copy of their advance decisions in their medical records.
- However no one specific document exists with which to but several charities have made appropriate documents available e.g.: The Alzheimer's Society.

The following document explains advance decisions in more detail and provides an example document: http://www.endoflifecareforadults.nhs.uk/eolc/files/NHS-EoLC_ADRT_Sep2008.pdf

Specific problem areas are covered here: http://www.endoflifecareforadults.nhs.uk/eolc/acpadrt.htm

Palliative care

As people near the end of life, care planning is less 'advanced care plan-ning' and becomes more immediate. The Gold Standards Framework (GSF) is specifically designed to identify these people.

GSF is a systematic evidence-based approach to optimizing the care for patients nearing the end of life delivered by generalist providers. It is concerned with helping people to live well until the end of life. It helps clinicians identify patients in the last years of life, assess their needs, symptoms and preferences and plan care on that basis.

Some definitions

Palliative care is the active care of patients whose disease is not respon-sive to curative treatment. It may be delivered by any health care pro-fessional and incorporates symptom control, and addresses social, psychological and spiritual problems. All health care professionals should be able to provide this with input from a specialist team needed only in complex cases. Palliative care can be provided in hospital, at home or in a hospice.

Terminal care is the care of a person in the last days or weeks before they die.

Specialist palliative care is delivered by those with specialist training in palliative care (McMillan nurses/Consultants in palliative medicine) and is useful for more difficult/complex cases.

The 'surprise question' should be asked of patients with chronic or life-threatening conditions: "Would I be surprised is this patient died in the next year?". This helps identify those who would benefit from the GSF. The key goals are:
1. Consistent high quality care
2. Alignment with patients' preferences
3. Pre-planning and anticipation of needs
4. Improved staff confidence and teamwork
5. More home based, less hospital based care

Once identified, these patients can be assessed and plans made to meet their needs using the '7 C's' approach:
- Communication
- Co-ordination
- Control of symptoms
- Continuity of care
- Continued learning
- Carer support
- Care of the dying pathway.

Patients should be regularly re-assessed (ideally as part of a regular MDT meeting as their needs will change as they move closer to the end of life). The GSF is running in three streams: primary care, care homes and other settings. It therefore has a wide scope which cannot be fully covered here. Further details can be found on the following website: http://www.goldstandardsframework.nhs.uk/.

Liverpool Care Pathway (LCP)

In the last hours and days of life, the LCP provides a standardised approach to patient care. It can be used anywhere that a person is dying and is designed to transfer the highest quality of care from the hospice movement to other clinical areas.

A patient expected to die in the next 72 hours can be placed on the pathway. It empowers the clinical team to focus on end of life care and stop all unnecessary observations, investigations and medications. It gives advice on prescribing appropriate palliative treatment and it facilitates discussions with families and patients. If a patient improves they can be moved off the pathway again.

The LCP is now well established in most care settings and a copy should be available to you. Alternatively you can use the following website: http://www.mcpcil.org.uk/liverpool-care-pathway/

Recommended reading

Department of Health (2008). End of life care strategy.
General Medical Council (2008). Patients and doctors making decisions together.
General Medical Council (2009). Confidentiality.

Chapter 14

Cardiovascular disease and mental health

Introduction

Older patients with cardiovascular disease not infrequently have mental health problems requiring treatment. Many of these treatments have cardiovascular side effects and it is often necessary to balance the risks and benefits of treatment. This short chapter covers some of the more important issues, namely depression, use of antipsychotics, and treatments for dementia.

Depression

- Depression in the elderly is frequently co-morbid with other physical disorders.
- The relationship between depression and cardiovascular disease is bidirectional, each increasing the risk of the other.
- Depression is strongly associated with coronary artery disease, heart failure, and myocardial infarction, and predicts a poorer prognosis in these conditions.
- Depression impacts significantly on health and social care systems.
- Depression impacts significantly on recovery and rehabilitation.
- Depression in the elderly patient with cardiovascular disease is often unrecognized and untreated.
- Depression may present atypically in the elderly: e.g. hypochondriasis, somatization, sudden onset of worry/irritability, and social withdrawal.
- Drugs used to treat cardiovascular conditions known to be depressogenic include β-blockers, calcium channel blockers, digoxin, angiotensin-converting enzyme (ACE) inhibitors, and methyldopa.
- Screening for depression in patients with cardiovascular disease is therefore important and recommended by the National Institute for Health and Clinical Excellence (NICE 2006). Screening tools for use in hospitals and the elderly are shown in Table 14.1. NICE recommends two screening questions. The Geriatric Depression Scale (GDS) is well validated and recommended by the British Geriatric Society and the Royal College of Physicians.

Table 14.1 Depression screening and rating scales

Scale	Comments
Brief Assessment Schedule Depression Cards (BASDEC)	Designed to screen medically ill elderly patients for depression in a ward setting. Patients need to be able to read and be cognitively intact
Evans Liverpool Depression Rating Scale (ELDRS)	Developed for use in physically unwell people in hospital setting
Geriatric Depression Scale (GDS)	Developed specifically for older adults and well validated in both 15 and 30 item formats as well as shorter 4/5 item format
Hospital Anxiety and Depression Scale (HADS)	Designed for use in general medical outpatients and screens for anxiety and depression separately
National Institute for Health and Clinical Excellence (NICE)	Recommends two screening questions: (1) During the last month, have you often been bothered by feeling down, depressed, or hopeless? (2) During the last month, have you often been bothered by having little interest or pleasure in doing things?
Cornell Scale for Depression in Dementia	A clinician-administered instrument for use in patients with dementia

Treatment of depression in elderly patients with cardiovascular disease

Treatment of depression is important as it impacts on the patients' physical and psychological function. However, caution is advised as all available antidepressants have important adverse effects that are more prominent in the elderly due to altered pharmacodynamics and pharmacokinetics and associated physical illness.

Important points to remember regarding treatment of depression in the elderly patient with cardiovascular disease are:

- Psychological treatments such as cognitive behavioural therapy, inter-personal therapy, psychodynamic psychotherapy, and problem solving treatment work as well in the elderly as in younger patients with mild to moderate depression. They are as effective as antidepressants so should be tried first as recommended by NICE. This is especially important in elderly patients with cardiovascular disease because of the considerable cardiovascular side effects of antidepressants.
- Avoid all antidepressants in first 2 months after myocardial infarction if possible.
- In patients who develop cardiovascular disease while on an antidepressant the need for treatment should be reviewed by an experienced physician as soon as possible and treatment withdrawn if appropriate. If treatment needs to continue it may be necessary to

switch to an agent with fewer cardiovascular side effects
(e.g. selective serotonin reuptake inhibitors (SSRIs) instead of a
tricyclic antidepressant (TCA) as described in this section).

- SSRIs are well tolerated and efficacious in the elderly and are
recommended as first line if drug treatment is necessary in patients
with cardiovascular disease. Start with low doses, especially in
patients with renal impairment. Side effects include hyponatraemia,
especially in patients with heart failure, increased risk of bleeding due
to interference with platelet function, acute confusion, and reduced
seizure threshold. SSRIs interact with warfarin, and citalopram and
escitalopram are the least likely to do this. If the patient fails to
respond or develops significant side effects, an alternative SSRI can
be tried before using venlafaxine.
- Venlafaxine, a dual action serotonin-norepinephrine reuptake inhibitor
(SNRI) is recommended as an alternative first-line treatment for
severe depression in elderly patients not responding or intolerant to
SSRIs. It can cause both postural hypotension and hypertension and
is contraindicated in poorly controlled hypertension (see Chapter 9
for guidance on blood pressure treatment), those at risk of significant
arrhythmias and within 2 months of acute myocardial infarction. Blood
pressure should be measured prior to starting treatment, at each dose
titration and 3–6 monthly thereafter.
- TCAs can cause postural hypotension which contributes to falls,
tachycardia (which can exacerbate angina), arrhythmias,
hyponatraemia, and reduced seizure threshold, and should be avoided
if possible in the elderly with cardiovascular disease. If a patient
develops heart disease while on a TCA the need for treatment should
be reviewed and the treatment withdrawn gradually. An SSRI can be
used as an alternative as already described in this section.
- Patients with psychotic depression may need addition treatment
with an antipsychotic but these should be used with caution in
cardiovascular disease (see Antipsychotics in elderly patients with
cardiovascular disease, p.308).
- Lithium can cause non-specific T wave changes on the
electrocardiogram (ECG). It is contraindicated in heart failure, renal
failure, and sick sinus syndrome.
- Aspirin increases the free plasma concentration of highly protein
bound drugs such as fluoxetine, paroxetine, sertraline, and sodium
valproate.
- Older people sometimes have negative preconceived ideas about
antidepressants and compliance is often poor, so education and
monitoring are important.

Antipsychotics in elderly patients with cardiovascular disease

- Antipsychotics are prescribed in the elderly to treat schizophrenia, psychotic depression, and neuropsychiatric symptoms in dementia (NICE 2004, 2006, 2009).
- There are major concerns regarding their use especially in cardiovascular disease.
- There are two major types, the older **conventional** antipsychotics and the newer **atypical** antipsychotics designed to increase efficacy and reduce side effects. Some examples are shown in Table 14.2.

Table 14.2 Examples of 'conventional' and 'atypical' antipsychotics

Conventional antipsychotics	Atypical antipsychotics
Chlorpromazine	Olanzapine
Haloperidol	Risperidone
Thioridazine	Quetiapine
Prochlorperazine	

- The newer drugs cause fewer extrapyramidal side effects and are less likely to cause neuroleptic malignant syndrome, but increase the risk of cardiovascular problems and blood dyscrasias. Both groups increase risk of obesity, blood glucose and serum lipid levels, oedema, and risk of stroke, sudden death, and falls.
- In elderly patients treated with antipsychotics (both conventional and atypical) there is 1.6–1.7-fold increased mortality. This is largely due to increased cardiovascular mortality presumed secondary to QT prolongation, arrhythmias, and sudden death.
- Most studies showing benefit of antipsychotics in treating neuropsychiatric symptoms in dementia are short term (up to 12 weeks).
- Studies have shown that psychological management can replace antipsychotic therapy without any appreciable worsening of neuropsychiatric symptoms, so we need to use these alternative approaches especially in elderly patients with cardiovascular disease.
- There is evidence that memantine and other anticholinesterase inhibitors (see later in this section) or antidepressants such as citalopram are effective alternatives for some neuropsychiatric symptoms so these used be tried first.
- The risks and benefits of prescribing antipsychotics to patients with neuropsychiatric manifestations of dementia need to be carefully balanced. These drugs should be used only if alternative strategies do not work and for a short period of time with regular review (preferably 3 monthly).
- Patients with dementia with Lewy bodies are at particular risk of adverse effects from antipsychotics.

- Patients who develop cardiovascular disease while on antipsychotic drug therapy should be reviewed at the earliest opportunity by an experienced clinician in mental health or health care for older people and the drug should be withdrawn if possible.
- When prescribing another medication to a patient receiving an antipsychotic it is especially important to be aware of the risk of drug interactions that may increase the risk of arrhythmia. This includes drugs that prolong the QT interval (Table 14.3), drugs causing electrolyte imbalance (Table 14.4), and drugs that inhibit or induce CYP450 metabolism, leading to increased or decreased plasma concentrations of the antipsychotic respectively (Table 14.5).

Table 14.3 Drugs that prolong QTc interval

Antipsychotics	Chlorpromazine, clozapine, haloperidol, quetiapine, risperidone, thioridazine
Antidepressants	Venlafaxine
Antiarrhythmics	Amiodarone, flecainide, sotalol, quinidine, procainamide, disopyramide
Antimicrobials	Clarithromycin, erythromycin, azithromycin
Others	Chloroquine, amantadine, lithium, methadone, tacrolimus

Table 14.4 Drugs that alter electrolyte balance

Diuretics
β_2-antagonists
Cisplatin
Laxatives
Corticosteroids
β-agonists

Table 14.5 Common medications that inhibit or induce CYP450 metabolism

Inhibit CYP450	Induce CYP450
CYP 1 A2: amiodarone, cimetidine, ciprofloxacin, paroxetine, interferon	CYP 1 A2: omeprazole, insulin, broccoli, Brussels sprouts, smoking
CYP 3A4, 5, 7: amiodarone, chloramphenicol, cimetidine, clarithromycin, erythromycin, grapefruit juice, fluconazole	CYP 3A4, 5,7: barbiturates, carbamazepine, phenytoin, pioglitazone, rifampicin, St John's wort, glucocorticoids
CYP 2D6: amiodarone, chlorphenamine, cimetidine, es/citalopram, fluoxetine, paroxetine, quinidine, ranitidine, sertraline	CYP 2D6: dexamethasone, rifampicin

Dementia and cardiovascular disease

- Dementia and cardiovascular disease both increase in prevalence with age, so many patients with cardiovascular disease will have or develop dementia as they age.
- The second-generation acetylcholinesterase (AChE) inhibitors, donepezil, rivastigmine, and galantamine introduced into clinical practice from 1997 are widely used for the symptomatic treatment of Alzheimer's disease.
- Concerns about the cardiovascular side effects of AChE inhibitors have led to wide variation in prescribing anticholinesterase inhibitors to patients with cardiovascular disease and patients who would benefit are often denied treatment because of over concern regarding the cardiovascular side effects.
- AChE inhibitors have a vagotonic effect on the heart and can cause sinus bradycardia and sinoatrial block, and can aggravate pre-existing sinus node disease and AV block. However, the risk of cardiovascular side effects is low (sinoatrial and AV block occur in <0.1%).
- There is no evidence that patients with pre-existing first-degree heart block are more likely to progress to second-degree or complete heart block while on treatment, and pre-morbid cardiovascular disease does not appear to be associated with a significantly increased incidence of cardiovascular adverse effects.
- Routine pretreatment ECGs are unnecessary and not useful at predicting cardiovascular adverse events; 24-hour cardiac monitoring is a relatively insensitive method of detecting arrhythmias, is poorly tolerated in patients with cognitive impairment and has high resource implications so is not routinely recommended.
- In patients prescribed an AChE inhibitor, pulse rate should be monitored prior to starting treatment and at 6-monthly intervals thereafter. If pulse rate is <50, even if asymptomatic we would advise withhold the drug and investigate. If unrelated to drug or a pacemaker is fitted the drug can be restarted.
- If a patient taking an AChE inhibitor presents with syncope or seizures an underlying cardiovascular cause should be suspected. The drug should be stopped and the patient referred for further investigation. If no causal relationship with the drug is found, or if a pacemaker is fitted, the drug may be restarted.
- Relative contraindications to the use of AChE inhibitors are sick sinus syndrome and cardiac conduction defects. My recommendation in these disorders would be a trial of therapy and if the patient has a good response careful monitoring at monthly intervals to detect symptomatic bradyarrhythmias requiring pacing would be appropriate. If a patient develops symptomatic bradycardia while on treatment and responding well, the drug should be temporarily withheld and a pacemaker inserted if appropriate.
- Extra vigilance and more frequent monitoring is advised in patients taking concurrent medications that reduce heart rate such as digoxin and β-blockers but there is no indication to discontinue these drugs prior to starting an AChE inhibitor.

- Dizziness is common in patients on AChE inhibitors (1–10%) and is usually mild and transient and unrelated to cardiovascular problems. The cause is often multifactorial, including infections, postural hypotension, and anaemia. If it associated with a relative bradycardia (pulse rate <60) or with falls, withhold the AChE inhibitor and consider referral to an elderly care physician for review. If symptoms are mild, continue treatment and monitor carefully.

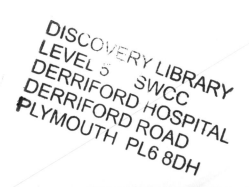

elines, references, and recommended reading

son IM, Ferrier IN, Baldwin RC, Cowen PJ, Howard L, Lewis G, et al. (2008) Evidence-based
delines for treating depressive disorders with antidepressants: A revision of the 2000 British
Association for Psychopharmacology guidelines. *J Psychopharmacol* **22**:343–96.

allard C, Hanney ML, Theodoulou M, Douglas S, McShane R, Kossakowski K, et al.; DART-AD
Investigators (2009) The dementia antipsychotic withdrawal trial (DART-AD): long-term
follow-up of a randomised placebo-controlled trial. *Lancet Neurol* **8**:151–7.

MacHale S (2002) Managing depression in physical illness. *Adv Psychiatr Treat* **8**:297–306.

National Institute for Health and Clinical Excellence (2004) Depression: management of
depression in primary and secondary care. Clinical guideline 23. London: National Institute for
Health and Clinical Excellence. Available from: www.nice.org.uk/cg23.

National Institute for Health and Clinical Excellence (2006) Dementia: Supporting people with
dementia and their carers in health and social care. Clinical guideline 42. London: National
Institute for Health and Clinical Excellence. Available from: www.nice.org.uk/cg42.

National Institute for Health and Clinical Excellence (2007) Donepezil, galantamine, rivastigmine
(review) and memantine for the treatment of Alzheimer's disease. Technology appraisal 111.
London: National Institute for Health and Clinical Excellence. Available from: www.nice.org.
uk/ta111.

National Institute for Health and Clinical Excellence (2009) Schizophrenia (update). Clinical
guideline 82. London: National Institute for Health and Clinical Excellence. Available from:
www.nice.org.uk/cg82.

Rowland JP et al. (2007) Cardiovascular monitoring with acetylcholinesterase inhibitors: a clinical
protocol. *Adv Psychiatr Treat* **13**:178–84.

Royal College of Psychiatrists (no date) Atypical antipsychotics and behavioural and psychiatric
symptoms of dementia. Prescribing update for old age psychiatrists. London: Royal College of
Psychiatrists. Available from: www.rcpsych.ac.uk/PDF/BPSD.pdf.

Wilson K, Mottram P, Sivanranthan A, Nightingale A (2001) Antidepressants versus placebo for
the depressed elderly. *Cochrane Database Syst Rev* (**2**):CD000561.

Index